Penguin Books

Alcoholism

Professor Neil Kessel received his medical education at Trinity College, Cambridge, and University College Hospital Medical School in London. His psychiatric training was at the University of London's Institute of Psychiatry and the Maudsley Hospital. From there he joined the scientific staff of the Medical Research Council and became Assistant Director of its unit for research on the epidemiology of psychiatric illness as well as being Consultant Psychiatrist at the Royal Infirmary of Edinburgh. Since 1965 he has held the Chair of Psychiatry at Manchester University. Professor Kessel has been both the Dean and the Postgraduate Dean of Medical Studies at Manchester. His principal research has been into suicide and self-poisoning acts, psychosomatic illness, psychiatric illness in general practice and alcoholism. Since 1974 he has been a member of the British General Medical Council and has served for long periods on the Health Education Council and on the Home Office Advisory Council for the misuse of drugs. For more than ten years he was Consultant Advisor on alcoholism to the Department of Health and Social Security and was also Chairman of its Advisory Committee on Alcoholism.

Professor Henry Walton was, until recently, Professor of Psychiatry at Edinburgh University, Director of the University Department of Psychiatry at the Western General Hospital and Consultant Psychiatrist at the Royal Edinburgh Hospital where he established the unit for treatment of alcoholism. He is now Professor of International Medical Education at the University of Edinburgh; President of the World Federation for Medical Education; President of the Association for Medical Education in Europe; and the editor of *Medical Education*. He is past-Chairman of the Society for Research into Higher Education and the Association for the Study of Medical Education. He formerly worked at the Maudsley Hospital and has taught and conducted research at the University of Cape Town and Columbia University in New York. As well as his work on alcoholism, Henry Walton has also published investigations into suicidal behaviour, psychological disturbance in old age, group psychotherapy, professional attitudes of medical practitioners and the effects of different teaching methods in training medical students and doctors.

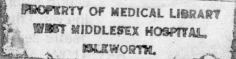

**This book is to be returned on or before
the last date stamped below.**

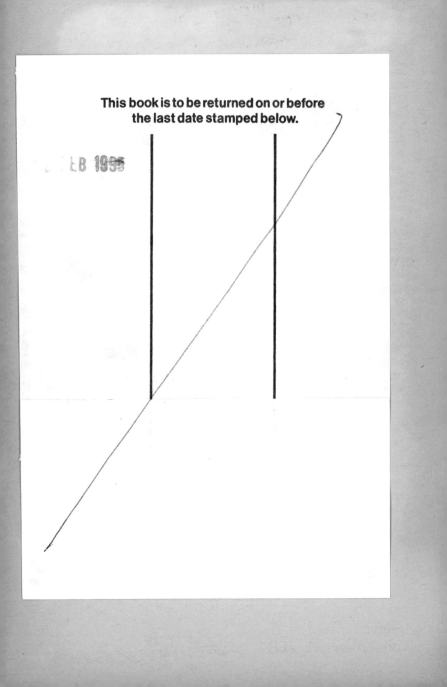

Alcoholism

Second Edition

Neil Kessel and Henry Walton

Penguin Books

Throughout this book we have made extensive
use of reports of the experiences of patients who
have been under our care, and we wish here to
acknowledge our debt to them.

PENGUIN BOOKS

Published by the Penguin Group
Penguin Books Ltd, 27 Wrights Lane, London W8 5TZ, England
Penguin Books USA Inc., 375 Hudson Street, New York, New York 10014, USA
Penguin Books Australia Ltd, Ringwood, Victoria, Australia
Penguin Books Canada Ltd, 10 Alcorn Avenue, Toronto, Ontario, Canada M4V 3B2
Penguin Books (NZ) Ltd, 182–190 Wairau Road, Auckland 10, New Zealand

Penguin Books Ltd, Registered Offices: Harmondsworth, Middlesex, England

First published in Pelican Books 1965
Reprinted with revisions 1967
Reprinted with revisions 1969
Second edition 1989
Reprinted in Penguin Books 1993
10 9 8 7 6 5 4 3 2 1

Printed in England by Clays Ltd, St Ives plc
Filmset in Linotron 202 Sabon

Contents

Foreword   vi

Preface   vii

1 What is an Alcoholic?   1

2 The Nature of Alcohol and its Intoxicating Effects   7

3 The Harmful Effects of Alcohol on the Body and Brain   13

4 Social Organization and Drinking   29

5 Personality Factors in Alcoholics   38

6 The Causes of Alcoholism   57

7 Varieties of Drinking Pattern   70

8 Stages in Being an Alcoholic   80

9 The Alcoholic's Family   93

10 Treatment   106

11 Results of Treatment   138

12 The Abstinent Alcoholic   145

13 Preventive Strategies and Public Health Aspects of Alcoholism   153

Notes   172

Index   177

Foreword

The first edition of this book appeared in 1965. It has since been reprinted many times but we have thought it right now to revise it completely. New knowledge about the causes of alcoholism and the development of new treatment methods have been the principal reasons for doing so, and the chapters covering these areas, together with that dealing with the results of treatment, have been totally recast and rewritten. Every one of the other chapters has been extensively altered so that the material presented is up to date.

Neil Kessel
Henry Walton
October 1987

Preface

The difference between having a drink and becoming drunk depends upon the quantity of alcohol taken. The amount needed to intoxicate will vary from person to person and from time to time, but anyone who drinks enough will get drunk. Between the drinker and the alcoholic there is another kind of difference. It cannot be measured in amounts of alcohol nor even be shortly defined. It depends upon intangibles, upon personality, upon opportunity, to some extent upon chance. Yet the steps from social to excessive drinking can be demarcated, and when harm results from the excessive drinking the drinker has become an alcoholic. Until they embarked upon this journey alcoholics were not obviously different from their fellows, although to the expert observer there might have been indications that they were predisposed.

We live in a society where it is customary to drink. With alcohol we offer hospitality and display our sociability. Though we frown on drunkards, we are suspicious of teetotallers. It is the abstainer who strikes us as abnormal. Over a glass we enjoy the company of old friends and make new ones, proclaim our loyalties, discuss affairs, negotiate and seal bargains. Repeated minimal intoxication is expected of our leading figures, soldiers, statesmen, businessmen, educators. This sort of drinking, open and well moderated, is, for the most part, harmless and conducive to good relationships.

In most cultures, social drinking is approved for the release which alcohol gives to an individual. At solemn ceremonies marking epochal events, birth, marriage and death, in religious ritual, in national celebration, in sporting victory and to mark the modest achievements of everyday life, alcohol has an honoured and accustomed place. Its merit is to help people join together to form groups. It reduces tension.

Strangers relax and mingle if alcohol is provided. Drinks are provided when for reasons of hospitality or business we want to create an atmosphere of warmth in a gathering of people who do not know each other well. Nor do we have to hide our intention, for guests welcome this social engineering. Drinks will make them socialize. Less apprehensive of their own failings, drinkers become less inclined to judge others critically. Society approves of regulated drinking because it oils the social wheels.

Individuals, for their part, have a double impetus to drink. They are complying with the social pattern and the effects of drinking are pleasurable. People do not drink only to attain particular mental or physical sensations. They are conforming to situations in which drinking is proper.

We are tolerant of the person who has a drink, or even a drink too many. Alcoholics also once drank moderately like this. What made them cross the line into alcoholism? Were the causes inexorably at work within them or in the environment and life circumstances? Physical, social and psychological factors have all to be considered. What is the course on which the alcoholic is now set? Where does the road lead and is there a way back? This book deals with all these questions.

The magnitude and seriousness of the illness of alcoholism are insufficiently appreciated. It is a grave disorder, often fatal. Its impact falls not only on the alcoholic but on a wide circle of family and friends. Its social reverberations affect accident and crime rates, absenteeism and unemployment. It is one of the largest causes of admissions to psychiatric units. Yet in many quarters, both medical and lay, this major threat to public health and welfare is not given serious consideration.

We shall deal in this book first with the physical and the psychological effects of alcoholism. Then, social and psychological factors conducive to alcoholism will be discussed, and the causes of alcoholism will be set out. Subsequent chapters will describe types of alcoholics and the progressive stages of the disease. Finally, we set out principles of treatment and prevention.

Chapter 1

What is an Alcoholic?

Three factors conspire to make alcoholism a difficult subject to grasp and to study. First, because many of the antics of the inebriated are comical, people often joke about alcoholics. What is in fact a considerable medical and social problem is thus eased out of serious consideration with a smile. Secondly, moral overtones colour our opinions, making it hard to amass information and arrive at proper judgements. Consequently, an objective assessment of the alcoholic is difficult. Someone who gets drunk at a party, or who drives a car when intoxicated, someone who spends so much on drink that the family's well-being is affected – with what words do we appraise him or her? Censure, blame, condemnation, disgust? Or do we despise, ostracize, punish? It is not easy to understand and even harder to sympathize or feel responsible. To study the problem of alcoholism scientifically it is necessary to free oneself completely of condemnatory attitudes. Moreover, such an approach is essential if anyone, doctor, helper or friend, is to be accepted by an alcoholic as competent to understand and help. Lastly, the problem of alcoholism is made more difficult by the lack of technical terms which are generally understood. What is an alcoholic? Without being adequately defined, the term is too readily applied to embrace everybody who drinks abnormally. Not all these are alcoholics. Furthermore, there are many different types of alcoholics and many varied patterns of alcoholism. Some define the alcoholic from the vantage point of the sufferer: they name as an alcoholic a person who recognizes drinking has to stop but cannot achieve this. Others have focused on the observable consequences of uncontrolled drinking: they define an alcoholic as a person whose drinking has caused increasing problems in his or her health, domestic or social life or work. Others emphasize the quantity of alcohol consumed and the pattern of the drinking habits: from their point of view alcoholics will drink greatly excessive amounts regularly and go on until they become helpless from drink.

A frame of reference is necessary if the subject is not to remain nebulous. We shall use the following terminology.

Some people are *teetotallers*.

Most people drink moderately. They may from time to time get drunk. These are *social drinkers*.

Some people drink excessively, though not necessarily in their own eyes; their excess may be shown either by the frequency with which they become intoxicated or by the social, economic or medical consequences of their continued intake of alcohol. These are *excessive drinkers*. Those excessive drinkers whose drinking gives rise to personal and social difficulties would do well not to equivocate but to recognize that alcohol lies at the root of their problem. Many excessive drinkers who have increasing difficulties arising from their use of alcohol may be in serious need of medical care and can respond to appropriate treatment. However, not all excessive drinkers are alcoholics, though probably the great majority of them proceed to this next stage.

Alcoholics are people with a disorder that can be defined in clinical terms and requires a proper regime of treatment. Most alcoholics are dependent upon alcohol. They used to be termed *alcohol addicts* but the word 'addiction' has come to be replaced by 'dependence'. The meaning is the same. They are unable spontaneously to give up drinking. Though they may go without a drink for a few days, or sometimes for even longer periods, there is a very great likelihood that they will revert. The greater the need to stop drinking the more difficult they find it to do so. Besides this characteristic of those dependent upon alcohol, that they cannot go for long without alcohol, they generally suffer from withdrawal symptoms – short-lived (though often serious) physical or mental ill-effects which supervene when drinking is temporarily halted for a few days or even hours.

Alcoholics may proceed to a stage where their brains or their bodies have been so harmed by alcohol that the effects persist even when they are not drinking. This stage may be reached by some excessive drinkers who had not manifested dependence. It is called *chronic alcoholism*. The term should only be applied when the body has been physically damaged by alcohol.

There are two essential elements to being an alcoholic. The first of these is *excessive drinking*, carrying the implication of repeated drinking. A single debauch does not, of itself, connote being an alcoholic. The second element is that *harm* results from the drinking. Unless there is harm someone may be an excessive drinker and may well be on the road to alcoholism, but he or she is not yet an alcoholic. Alcoholic harms may be physical, psychological or social. They may occur in any one of these spheres or in more than one. One important harm is *dependence* upon alcohol. The World Health Organization, in its International Classification of Diseases, now employs the term 'alcohol dependence syndrome' but stresses that 'not every individual who experiences impairment or disability related to alcohol consumption will be suffering from alcohol dependence'.

We thus define an alcoholic as a person who: (1) repeatedly drinks excessive quantities of alcohol; and (2) suffers an alcoholic harm.

To classify particular drinkers may not be easy, yet it is essential if they are to be helped. We cannot properly proceed until we know whether they are social drinkers, excessive drinkers, excessive drinkers with problems, alcohol dependent or have reached the further stage of chronic alcoholism. We need, in short, to know whether they are harmed, and, if so, what the particular harms are.

Dependence upon alcohol is different from dependence on other dangerous drugs, such as opium, heroin, and cocaine. In the first place, dependence on alcohol is far more accepted by society, because drinking is to a large extent socially condoned. Secondly, people dependent upon the other drugs may work up to a dose greatly exceeding that which would be fatal to an ordinary person; those dependent on alcohol do not go on increasing their intake in the same way. The level of acquired tolerance is much less. Although habituated alcoholics are not as affected by alcohol as novice drinkers, they do not need to drink greatly increased quantities to continue to get the desired effect. When people dependent on drugs stop taking them they experience a craving: physiological changes set up a subjective need for more of the drug. They also develop withdrawal symptoms which are promptly alleviated by another single dose. The alcoholic may be able to abstain for quite long periods without craving, particularly if in a hospital or other institution.

If withdrawal effects occur, they are not at once abolished by a single further dose of drink. This fact accounts for the craving being much less imperative than it is following the withdrawal of most dangerous drugs. The term *dependence* is appropriate to alcoholics, however, in one very important sense: even though they may not need to take it constantly, i.e. they may not be physically dependent, alcoholics have to rely upon alcohol, from time to time if not continuously. With its aid they can face a problem, their family and themselves. The alcoholic is dependent upon alcohol to function efficiently as a social being. It is the irony of this which makes alcoholism into a problem, for the very stuff which alcoholics rely on in order to function has the inexorable physiological effect of impairing function.

To resolve this situation, to help the alcoholics to be able to conduct their lives without alcohol, is called 'treatment'. So we can now understand, even though we need not agree with every aspect of it, the pioneering World Health Organization's definition[1] of the alcoholic:

> Alcoholics are those excessive drinkers whose dependence on alcohol has attained such a degree that they show a noticeable mental disturbance or an interference with their mental and bodily health, their interpersonal relations and their smooth social and economic functioning; or who show the prodromal signs of such developments. They therefore require treatment.

'Treatment' suggests something which only doctors can give.

But the help which alcoholics require should be given by all those associated with them: family, friends and employers as well as social agencies, members of the other health professions and doctors. Directly or indirectly, alcoholism is everyone's concern; and it is a growing problem. In Chapter 13 we discuss in more detail its extent, and the extent of its several harms.

The fact that alcoholism is an illness should be more generally appreciated in Britain both by the public and by doctors. In 1935 the American Medical Association passed a resolution which stated that 'Alcoholics are valid patients'. This is the counterpart of WHO's 'They therefore deserve treatment'. In Britain many doctors and others responsible for organizing health services are still reluctant to accept this.

Alcoholism also poses social problems both for the community and for the individual alcoholics and their families. In most cities there are to be found depressed areas where alcoholics congregate, limbos where they eke out poverty-stricken, degenerate, sometimes psychotic existences. Alcoholism leads to absenteeism and unemployment, debt, crime, social decline and sometimes child neglect.

There are other social ills which, if they cannot directly be laid at the door of alcoholism, are certainly related to it. There is evidence that alcoholics swell the number of arrests for drunkenness, particularly of young adults, and that they are responsible for many road accidents due to drinking. There has also been a great increase, both in drinking and in alcoholism, amongst women.

Whether an alcoholic is viewed as a medical or as a social problem will profoundly affect the future course of the disorder. Where alcoholics are dealt with by the courts they may possibly spend time in prison in a custodial atmosphere that is not directed at rehabilitation. Where medical treatment is available and doctors are prepared to accept responsibility for the management of the condition, the institution to which the alcoholic is admitted (if indeed admission is required) is more likely to be a hospital. The measures adopted will be therapeutic, designed to foster self-respect and sustain the resolve to overcome the disability. Today in Britain each method is applied, but the disposal generally depends not upon individual needs but on the relatively trivial circumstances that bring alcoholics to the notice of one or other service. Anyone responsible for dealing with an alcoholic ought to obtain all the information available, medical and social, and reflect seriously whether the allocation decided upon fits the individual requirements.

Recently there has been a tendency to try to replace the words 'alcoholic' and 'alcoholism' by the terms 'problem drinkers' and 'alcohol-related disabilities'. We have not followed this path. In fact these terms have been invented to soften the blow and to make it easier for people to accept that they have to face up to the realities of their situation. But the situation is that they are alcoholics and indeed they are not going to be helped by watered-down phraseology that hides the truth. Similarly, the term 'alcohol-related disabilities' means no more than harms resulting from excessive drinking, and alcoholism means precisely that. Non-medical personnel have particularly seized on such terminology because they believe that its acceptance would result in a de-medicalization of alcoholism. As will be seen, however, in Chapter 10, calling someone an alcoholic and labelling the problem as alcoholism does not force us to regard each sufferer as medically ill, nor do we in any way urge that treatment of alcoholics has to be a medical matter. We do, however, insist that they require a detailed medical examination as part of their assessment.

Chapter 2

The Nature of Alcohol and its Intoxicating Effects

The chemist recognizes many different alcohols, but the one we drink is called ethyl alcohol. Carbon, hydrogen and oxygen are its only chemical elements, existing in a simple combination to form a colourless liquid. Two linked atoms of carbon have five hydrogen atoms attached to form the ethyl radical. A hydroxyl (or alcohol) group completes the chemical molecule. In the diagram, C, H and O stand for single atoms of carbon, hydrogen and oxygen; OH denotes the hydroxyl group.

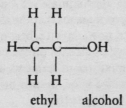

ethyl   alcohol

Other alcohols can be made by adding or subtracting carbon and hydrogen atoms, but only the ethyl variety has the conventional effects of alcohol as we know them, and only ethyl alcohol is safe to consume. Alcohol can be prepared easily from many plants and has been known to man from earliest times all over the world.

Although the chemist can make it from its basic constituents, the alcohol we drink comes from fermentation by yeast of sugars that occur naturally in plants. The drinks produced by such fermentation, beer from barley, wine from grapes and cider from apples, are relatively weak in alcohol. Beer usually contains between 2·5 and 4·5 per cent alcohol by volume, though strong beers may have higher proportions. Ciders are roughly of comparable strength. Most wines contain between 10 per cent and 12 per cent alcohol.

The strength of spirits is much greater, the extra concentration being produced by distillation. In Britain they generally contain between 30 per cent and 40 per cent of alcohol, more in the United States of America. In this country, 40 per cent is the usual strength for gin and whisky (though some malt whiskies are stronger). Rum, brandy and vodka are of similar but more variable strength. The strength of liqueurs varies widely. The strength of spirits may be recorded as so many 'degrees proof'. This harks back to an old measure of the concentration of alcohol devised by the early distillers. Gunpowder mixed with water will not ignite, but mixed with alcohol it will. If mixtures of alcohol and water are tried it is found that a combination of half alcohol, half water will allow the gunpowder to ignite but weaker concentrations of alcohol will not. The strength of the spirit used to be *proved* in this way. Proof spirit contains approximately 57 per cent of alcohol by volume; 70 degrees proof means that the alcohol content is about 40 per cent. However, nowadays it is becoming increasingly usual to state the percentage of alcohol on the bottle label.

Some drinks are mixtures of ferments and distillates. Sherry, for instance, is a fortified wine, brandy being added to bring the alcohol strength up to 20 per cent.

No matter what beverage is drunk, the alcoholic effect depends on the amount of alcohol consumed and not on the colouring, flavouring, or any other constituents.

Alcohol exerts, according to its strength, an effect on the lining of the mouth, the oesophagus, the stomach and the upper part of the intestines. In the mouth this is experienced as a burning sensation, pleasant or slightly painful. The expression 'That hits the spot!' well describes the stinging and the satisfying effects of a glass of spirits quickly drunk. From the stomach and intestines the alcohol is absorbed into the bloodstream and passes rapidly into all the tissues and fluids of the body. Gradually it is destroyed by oxidation, principally in the liver, and it is eventually broken down into carbon dioxide and water. A small quantity, perhaps 2 per cent, escapes this process and is excreted in the urine and in the breath. The amount of alcohol breathed out is very small indeed, but is sufficient to permit the use of breath tests to detect the concentration of alcohol in the body. The smell on a drinker's breath is imparted chiefly by other volatile constituents of drinks and is no index of the extent of intoxication. The rate at which alcohol is oxidized is independent of the concentration in the body; because the maximum rate is quickly reached it follows that it will take much longer for someone who has drunk very heavily to return to normal than it does for a moderate drinker. Four ounces of whisky or four pints of beer might take four or five hours to be oxidized, and if the amount drunk is doubled it would take twice as long. For this reason people who drink slowly but continuously, though they may appear less incapable, take as long to recover from drinking as those who have absorbed a similar quantity rapidly.

The effects of alcohol which we experience as intoxication, or getting drunk, are due to its action upon the nervous system, but changes also occur elsewhere in the body. The heart rate may rise a little, and there is an increased flow in the blood vessels resulting in flushing and a warm sensation in the skin. The rate of urine production rises, chiefly as a consequence of the amount of fluid that is drunk but also because alcohol influences the pituitary gland which controls the rate of urine formation.

Alcohol is a food. As a provider of calories it must, in Britain, be one of the most expensive, and certainly the most extensively taxed. It is a carbohydrate, and because of its rapid absorption from the stomach it is a quick source of energy. However, this energy cannot be used efficiently because of the incoordinating and intoxicating effects of alcohol. Only the self-deceiving can believe they are doing something dietetically useful by drinking.

Alcohol is claimed to be an aphrodisiac and to promote sexual function. It may stimulate desire, and the shy or cautious person may, under its influence, be able to make love because inhibitions, fears or scruples have been lessened. However, this is a psychological effect. Upon potency alcohol exerts a dampening action.

Alcohol reduces the activity of the nervous system. All its functions are depressed. How is it, therefore, that alcohol has come to be widely thought of as a stimulant? Unless we can resolve this paradox we shall never understand the use of alcohol by man.

Let us marshal the evidence for stating so categorically that it depresses activity in the nervous system. On the physical side it numbs like an anaesthetic so that people may fall when drunk and not appreciate that they have hurt themselves; it may send one to sleep; it may even make one unconscious. It alters the rhythm of brain activity, as can be seen when this is recorded electrically from the head. Even in small amounts it affects speech and balance and impairs judgement. After a few drinks our ability to react promptly to a changing situation or an emergency is reduced, so that we ought not to drive a vehicle. We may be able to cope with an empty road or usual traffic, but if a car were to approach unexpectedly or someone step off the kerb suddenly we could not make the appropriate response quickly enough to prevent the accident.

In ordinary social intercourse, at a party for instance, we can no longer so finely or so rapidly assess what it is proper for us to say or to keep silent about. Here lies the explanation of the paradox. The first thing to be depressed is the power of restraint. The inhibition of our actions or our wishes, which we all of us adopt in order to get on with our fellows, is the product of the highest mental processes, and it is these that are impaired first. When the curb we normally place on our instinctual urges goes, unguarded behaviour comes to the fore, and these released impulses are forcefully expressed, giving the impression of stimulation. The solitary become gregarious, shy people find themselves loquacious and the fearful may become foolhardy. Self-critical people can treat themselves kindly, the sexually inhibited dare to be amorous. At first the increased talk and activity sets up smiles, gaiety, even boisterousness, but generally we retain enough self-control to keep these within bounds. Most social drinking never proceeds further than this, and the atmosphere produced may indeed be stimulating. It is also infectious. If one or two members of a party decide not to drink because they will be driving home, they generally find that the communal laughter, affection and good spirits rub off onto them as well, so that they are able to share in the general feeling of well-being.

Sometimes, however, the drinking facilitates a group mood of dejection or anger, and groups of people have had their passions so inflamed by alcohol that they carried out cruel, senseless, irrevocable actions from which, if the highest mental processses were functioning intact, each individual would recoil with disgust. This, of course, is the extreme, but the morning-after reaction sometimes contains a sense of amazement and shame that one could have done the things one did so carelessly the night before. One effect of drinking in a social setting is that individual characteristics and restraints are lessened, and group, one might almost say herd, instincts assume predominance.

These changes, which the physician and the physiologist call depression of the nervous system, begin with the first drink. There is not a level below which one can drink without any noticeable change but above which one is affected. Fine tests of discriminatation, memory and driving skills all show that the impairment begins with the beginning of drinking and advances steadily with the continuation of drinking. We know too that a vicious circle is set up: the more we drink, the more our faculties and our judgement are lost, and consequently the less we appreciate this falling off of our skills. It is this which allows clearly incapable people to believe they are fit to drive. In one experiment,[2] bus drivers, after drinking different amounts, were asked to judge whether they could get their buses between two movable posts. As they drank more and more they became less accurate in deciding, but more certain that they were right. This is one reason why it is impossible to state an amount of drink or blood concentration of alcohol below which it is all right to drive. For legal purposes an arbitrary level may have to be fixed, but the truth is that some impairment occurs with any drinking, one small whisky, one glass of beer. The drinkers themselves are not in a good position to decide whether it is safe for them to drive.

During a single episode of drinking, certain levels of alcohol concentration in the blood will be achieved, these levels increasing as further drinking takes place. Later on, as the drinker sobers up, the blood concentration will again pass through these levels as it falls. If we make psychological observations at two points in time when blood concentration is the same, one when it is rising and one when it is falling, we observe that the drinker's performance is better on the later occasion. The drinker's nervous system has in some measure accommodated to the body's alcohol. Neither the amount that is drunk nor the blood alcohol level, therefore, can be an absolute guide to a person's capabilities.

Another reason why it is dangerous to lay down safe amounts to drink is that increased tolerance occurs in drinkers. This phenomenon explains why not all people who drink the same amount become equally intoxicated. Different people are differently affected by the same intake of alcohol. Some have more tolerance than others; that is to say, their efficiency is less impaired. Individuals develop increased tolerance during the course of their drinking careers; at the outset they will be much more affected by, say, six whiskies than they will be later on. Still later, especially if they fall sick or are undernourished, tolerance may again decline. This accounts for the distressing experience of many advanced alcoholics that suddenly they become much more disorganized by an amount of drink which they had previously thought they could handle without difficulty.

During the process of acquiring tolerance the cells of the body become seasoned to alcohol so that a given concentration affects them less than it used to. How this tolerance develops is not known. It has nothing to do with the rate of absorption, metabolism or excretion of alcohol; but the cells of the body, in particular those of the brain, get used to functioning in the presence of higher concentration of alcohol than they could tolerate before.

Nevertheless, although these factors tell us not to describe any amount of drink as 'safe', they do let us recommend levels that are unsafe. Unfortunately, these levels, which can be found on p. 161, have come to be known as 'safe limits'. We hope it will be clear that, although it can be useful to have such guides in terms of quantity and frequency of drinking, they need to be used in the context of knowing what one's individual reactions are.

Chapter 3

The Harmful Effects of Alcohol on the Body and Brain

Looking at a stranger it is most unlikely that you could identify them as an alcoholic from their appearance alone. It is easy to tell that a person is drunk but not that anyone is a habitual drinker. Yet continued excessive drinking does produce bodily changes, and these in turn result in illnesses both physical and mental.

From the physical standpoint the most serious consequence of alcoholism is *malnutrition*. This arises in two ways. Chronic alcoholics do not eat enough, and what they do eat does not nourish them as well as it should. Alcoholics do not eat enough partly because earnings may be small but also because they redistribute their spending so as to buy more drink and consequently less food. Drinking becomes a more pressing necessity than eating. Frequently, alcoholics are forced to fend for themselves because spouse and relations have left. The desire to cook and the facilities to do it may both be inadequate, so recourse is had to the expensive practice of buying prepared foods. The diet may then be excessively starchy and deficient in protein. If they take their food in pubs so as to be able to drink at the same time, they subsist chiefly on rolls, potato crisps, and occasional sausages. The high price of food in public houses constitutes a further economic setback. They will get enough in sheer calories, however, because of the alcohol. Besides the lack of protein, such a diet tends to be *deficient in vitamins*, particularly in vitamin B.

These considerations apply more to the poor than to the rich alcoholic, but even wealthy habitual drinkers are likely to suffer from missed meals and from self-induced restrictions of diet because the appetite has gone. The alcoholic prefers to forgo solid for liquid refreshment.

The alcoholic's lack of appetite (*anorexia*) is often accompanied by morning nausea which leads to giving up breakfast; during the day the constant supply of alcoholic calories between meals reduces feelings of hunger, and the effect of an inflamed stomach (*gastritis*) or of a diseased liver (*cirrhosis*) will be to produce further anorexia. These factors, independently or in concert, may result in even more serious *nutritional deficiency*, since food may not be properly absorbed from the intestines or metabolized for the body's use. We arrive at the position where malnutrition itself contributes to cirrhosis of the liver, and this, in its turn, results in further malnutrition. Once the alcoholic reaches a certain stage of physical change therefore, further decline is generally rapid.

Chronic alcoholism is the commonest cause of liver disease. The alcohol itself exerts a direct toxic effect on the liver cells, and the poor absorption of food from the intestine, coupled with an inadequate diet, together produce an insufficiency of some substances essential to the liver's good repair. Although the liver disease may in its early stages be mild and reversible, if it continues undetected it readily progresses to the severe form, which is called cirrhosis because of the scarring and hardening which the liver undergoes. The chief clinical features are a feeling of illness ('liverishness' is the name given to its mild form), flatulence, anorexia and sallowness of the skin. About a third of all sufferers develop *jaundice*. Vomiting of blood and the accumulation of fluid in the abdomen may both occur late in the disease, which kills about half of those afflicted with it. Women are more vulnerable than men to developing cirrhosis at lower levels of drinking.

Before cirrhosis develops, the alcoholic is likely to suffer fairly severely from gastritis. Indeed some purely social drinkers are affected by this condition to such an extent that the pain and flatulence actually stop them from drinking any further. The inflammation of the stomach from which the condition gets its name is caused directly by the irritant property of strong drinks: spirits cause it more than beer or wine. The blood-vessels of the stomach become dilated and the whole lining is covered in mucus. In addition, the stomach ceases to contract normally but distends, giving rise to discomfort and flatulence. Gastritis is the simplest of all the alcoholic conditions to cure. It goes away quickly once drinking stops.

The pancreas is another organ of digestion, situated behind the stomach and responsible for producing a number of digestive juices. It also makes insulin. When it is attacked by alcohol, therefore, some patients have a further disability of digestion and a few develop diabetes – usually mildly. However, the chief effect of chronic inflammation of the pancreas caused by alcohol is a continuous severe pain felt in the abdomen or back. The alcoholic origin of the condition often goes unrecognized, yet alcoholism is a frequent cause of *pancreatitis*.

Other physical illnesses brought about by chronic alcoholism are borne by the nervous system. An important cause is malnutrition, resulting in a deficiency of one or more of the B vitamins. This is responsible for a common condition, *peripheral neuritis*. The nerve fibres bear the brunt of this condition, and the longer nerves, those which stretch all the way from the spinal column to the ends of the limbs, are the most involved. Hence the neuritis is 'peripheral'. It mainly affects the toes and the feet, the fingers and the hands, beginning with a sensation of tingling, pins and needles, and progressing to numbness. Because the nerves to the skin are affected, the sufferers cannot finely assess what they are touching and may not know that there is anything in their hand if they do not look. Ups and downs of the ground surface may not be appreciated, and they feel that they are all the time walking not on a firm surface but on cotton wool. In a later stage the nerves to the joints become damaged so that the patient may no longer know the position of feet or hands. Consequently they keep falling. The sensory nerves are affected earlier than those responsible for muscular movement, but as the condition progresses weakness develops, first in the extremities and later spreading towards the trunk. Peripheral neuritis may require treatment in bed. Vitamin B therapy is necessary and it may be many months before recovery is complete.

Alcoholism often produces a characteristic type of change in the red blood cells that tells an expert the cause. Indeed, large red blood cells without anaemia are considered by many to be virtually diagnostic of alcoholism and therefore of some use as a screening test for alcoholism.

These physical ravages of alcoholism occur, for obvious reasons, late in its course. If treatment is not commenced and vigorously carried out, the patient is likely to pursue a progressive downhill course towards invalidism and death. Fortunately, medical attention can no longer be evaded, and, provided that the physician does not enter into a covert conspiracy with the patient to gloss over the true nature of the condition, the alcoholic may be persuaded into accepting treatment to give up drinking.

As we will emphasize later, the great tragedy is that many doctors persistently disregard the alcoholism, perceiving only its complications as treatable. When this neglect of the underlying cause occurs, then even if the physical symptoms can be made to remit, they will recur should the resolve to stop drinking not continue. This is likely to happen if treatment aimed at combating the alcoholism itself is not applied.

The *hangover* experienced by alcholics differs somewhat from the unpleasant sensation that many non-alcoholics must have experienced and called by the same name. It consists of a time-limited group of symptoms of variable severity occurring when drinking is interrupted. Psychological symptoms are tension, anxiety, dejection, impoverished thinking, diminished drive, and asociability; sleep disorder is usual and nausea can also occur. In fact, the hangover can be so awful that alcoholics who regularly go 'on the wagon' are further cast down by the certainty that the whole scenario, brief though it may be, will endlessly recur. The hangover's causes are complex and not completely known, but dehydration is an important aspect.

Withdrawal symptoms are brought about by stopping drinking or by a sudden reduction in the amount taken. In consequence a drop in the concentration of alcohol in the blood occurs. Heavy drinkers of some years' duration, who have maintained a very high alcohol intake continuously for some days or weeks before stopping, are sensitive to this reduction in concentration and develop symptoms. The same symptoms which follow alcohol withdrawal can also be produced by the sudden cutting off of sleeping tablets by anyone who has been taking heavy doses for some time. Because of this similarity in withdrawal symptoms, alcohol and sedative drugs are classified in the same group of dependence-forming substances.

Symptoms occur at any time from a few hours to a few days after stopping drinking. Milder symptoms begin first; delirium tremens, the most severe, begins later. The earliest and commonest withdrawal state is *acute tremulousness*. This is what physicians call it, but alcoholics know it as 'the shakes'. It follows so soon upon reduction in heavy drinking that it may in fact come on before drinking has completely stopped. Fall in alcohol concentration, not necessarily zero concentration, brings it about. Usually it takes a few hours to develop, and consequently many alcoholics are affected by it each morning: 'When I wake up I have to take a drink to steady myself' is a common complaint. In this state the alcoholic is agitated, jumpy and easily startled. The principal feature is gross shaking of the hands, made worse when trying to do anything with them. Sometimes there is a feeling of being shaky inside. There is anxiety, physical restlessness and a feeling of weakness. Agitation and tremor can reach such a degree that the person may not be able to sit still, to dress or to pour out a drink without spilling it. The condition disappears fairly rapidly, though not at once, when drink is taken; without alcohol it may persist for a week or more. A quarter of those who suffer moderate or severe attacks have accompanying hallucinations. These are usually short-lived and may only be admitted to after they have ceased to be experienced. Then the alcoholic tells about a vivid nightmare which was difficult to disentangle from reality. The hallucinations may be visual or auditory. Things around may appear distorted in shape; shadows seem to be real and to move. Shouting or snatches of music may be heard and the innocent remarks of bystanders may be misinterpreted, whether addressed to the alcoholic or not. When examined at this time, especially if in the unfamiliar surroundings of a hospital or police station, the alcoholic may not be sure where he or she is and may be unaware of the time of day or the day of the week. This is called disorientation.

Delirium tremens is one of the most dramatic conditions in the whole calendar of medicine. To the observer there is a rapidly changing picture of bewildering, disordered mental activity. For the sufferer every conscious moment is one of extreme fear. Fear, agitation and great distractibility are dominant features; disorientation and hallucinations are the most vivid. Delirium tremens – DTs – generally begins two to five days after stopping very heavy drinking. It may be the first manifestation, though frequently the state of tremulousness passes imperceptibly into it. There have usually been at least ten years of excessive drinking before the first attack.

The symptoms are florid; there is great restlessness and agitation. In the hospital ward the patient, despite being weak, may have to be restrained by two or more people before being got into bed. Never still, tossing and turning restlessly, constantly engaged in conversation, switching from person to person and from subject to subject at the smallest stimulus, they are noisy, frequently shouting out greetings or warnings to passers by. The hands, shaking wildly, clutch at the bedclothes; continuously the delirious patient tries to pick from them imaginary objects, shining coins, burning cigarettes, playing cards, or bed bugs. A prey to ever-changing visual hallucinations, the alcoholic may shield his face from perceived menacing attacking objects, animals or men. At any moment the attention can be distracted by a chance gesture or remark made by someone nearby. The pupils of the eyes are dilated and the ceaseless exertion gives rise to rapid pulse and sometimes a fever.

The patient is completely disoriented and may not recognize the surroundings, the time of day, the date or even the month. Someone experiencing delirium tremens misidentifies people, thinking for instance that the nurse is a waitress, at one moment failing to recognize familiar people, at another greeting strangers as old friends, calling them by name and, if induced to do so, inventing the circumstances of their last meeting. They are intensely suggestible and readily respond to the promptings of others so that, for example, they may be induced to tell the time from a blank circle if told that it is a clock. There is a state of complete confusion.

The prevailing mood is one of frightful apprehension, which

arises predominantly from misperception and misrepresentation of the surroundings. The sufferer feels that he or she is being threatened from all sides and may fight to ward off attackers. The mind reacts in this way because the ego, the executive part of the self, cannot perform its functions when there is acute disorganization of the brain. The alcoholic has been coping with the sensed disapproval of other people for a long time and in the confused state now acts on fears and suspicions which are normally repressed.

There is no need to inquire about hallucinations: their presence is only too apparent. Patients respond to imaginary voices and react to imagined sights. They see, in particular, rapidly moving small objects. Rats and mice are traditionally described, but often the animals are far more threatening – big black flies buzzing at the face, cats coming to claw at the patient. Sometimes the hallucinations are more bizarre: 'Zip-fastening suitcases biting at my legs,' said one patient. Sometimes the fear changes to resignation: 'I know you're going to kill me: get on with it.' Sometimes there are moments of bonhomous joviality when the patient will offer 'drinks all round'; but it is not long before fear reasserts itself. No words can do justice to the picture of fully developed delirium tremens during the hours or days before the patient falls exhausted into a deep sleep. From this they generally emerge little the worse, though feeling weak and tired and with memory for the recent events mercifully blunted.

Unchecked, the condition usually takes three or more days to run its course, but fortunately it can now be considerably modified by drugs. Deaths still occur, largely as a result of other illnesses present at the same time. Since the delirium is a withdrawal reaction we have to ask why the drinking was stopped. Usually this is because something made it impossible for the alcoholic to keep up his supply. Often it is being admitted to hospital with an illness, such as pneumonia, or with an injury following an accident that interrupts alcohol intake. Unless it is realized that the person is an alcoholic and, therefore, the possibility of developing delirium tremens is anticipated, the subsequent enforced withdrawal of alcohol will not be compensated for by appropriate medication. Three days or so later the physician or surgeon will be presented with a case of delirium tremens. However, if the possibility is borne in mind, an attack can be prevented or rapidly checked.

Alcoholic epilepsy, when it occurs, follows within a day or two of stopping drinking. Fits can be provoked in anybody given a sufficient stimulus, but the effect of alcohol withdrawal is to increase the susceptibility of the brain to undergo spontaneous electrical discharges resulting in fits. There may be single seizures or bursts. They are generally major convulsions in which consciousness is lost, and they have to be managed in the same way as other forms of symptomatic epilepsy.

The knowledge that these states, alcoholic tremulousness, alcoholic epilepsy and delirium tremens, are phenomena resulting from alcoholic withdrawal has been gained by two decisive research procedures: first, meticulous observation of the timing of their onset in relation to the end of drinking, and secondly, the production of similar states following the sudden withdrawal of sedatives.

So far we have discussed the damage done to the body by excessive drinking. We must now turn to abnormal mental states which arise from the effects on the brain of prolonged excessive intake. Mental symptoms of chronic alcoholism may be caused in either of two ways: from vitamin deficiency or from destruction of brain cells.

Chronic alcoholics are likely to be deficient in vitamin B. This lack causes mental disorders which are not the result simply of alcohol withdrawal. One is a severe disturbance of memory. In this state consciousness is not impaired and there is no confusion. The condition is commonly first noticed when an attack of delirium tremens is ending, but it is not otherwise related to it. The memory loss is selective and is best described in the account given in 1877 by the Russian psychiatrist Korsakov, by whose name the *amnestic syndrome* has long been called:

> In these cases disorder of memory manifests itself in the form of a remarkably peculiar amnesia (memory loss) in which the memory of

recent events is disturbed, whereas long past events remain remembered quite well. Mostly the amnesia of this particular type develops following prodromal agitation with confusion. This agitation lasts several days, and then the patient becomes calm again. His consciousness clears; he appears to be in better possession of his faculties; he receives information correctly, yet his memory remains deeply affected . . . On first contact with the patient one may not note the presence of psychiatric disorder. The patient impresses one as in possession of all his faculties; he reasons perfectly well, makes correct deductions from given propositions, jokes, plays chess or a game of cards; in short, comports himself as a psychically normal person. Only after a long conversation one may note that the patient confuses events, that he remembers absolutely nothing of what happens around him. He does not remember whether he had his dinner, or whether he got out of bed. At times he forgets what occurred just an instant ago. You have come into his room, conversed with him, and stepped out for a moment. You return, and the patient has no recollection that you have talked to him a moment ago. Persons whom the patient learns to know only in the course of the disease, e.g. his doctor or nurse, he cannot remember, and he assures them that he sees them for the first time. However, he remembers quite accurately past events which occurred before the illness.

It is almost unbelievable how short-lived the patient's memory can be. One patient awoke each morning believing he had been admitted to hospital during the previous night. A patient who was a stockbroker, after weeks in the ward, still required to read the names at the foot of each bed in order to find his own when returning from the toilet. Yet so well were his other faculties preserved that he had lost a fortune over the past few months without anyone realizing he was ill. He had forgotten to make the investment changes that his clients had ordered. To compensate for the memory loss the patient may confabulate, that is, invent circumstances to fill in the gaps in his memory and try to cover them up. The doctor can readily induce such confabulations by suggestion. In addition to the memory loss, or perhaps because of it, intelligence suffers. Problem-solving in both actual life and in psychological testing is not so well performed as previously. Once the amnestic syndrome has developed it is not possible to reverse it completely, though considerable recovery of memory may slowly occur with correct medication.

In another condition, *Wernicke's encephalopathy*, there is great difficulty in concentrating and slowness in answering questions although consciousness is full. It is frequently but not invariably associated with a memory loss of the Korsakov type. There is also a paralysis of some of the movements of the eyeballs and frequently a disturbance of gait and balance. This condition is associated with pathological changes in particular areas in the base of the brain, due to deficiency of vitamin B.

A number of chronic alcoholics show evidence of a continuing decline in intelligence as their drinking years progress. This is know as *alcoholic dementia*. Insidiously there is a falling off in their intellectual ability. They become less perceptive of what goes on around them, less capable of subtle evaluation of their experiences, and they are handicapped in their ability to convey their meaning to others. New and complicated tasks are harder to perform and consequently less inviting; they become duller. This is gradually perceived by their relatives and associates but is incorrectly thought of as a behaviour change rather than as evidence of intellectual loss. Psychological tests reveal the true nature of this state because they provide evidence of organic impairment of intelligence. The condition is due to destruction of brain cells. Brain scanning, a recent investigative technique that provides images of the brain, reveals there is loss of brain tissue. Moreover, this investigation has shown that the loss of brain tissue begins earlier in the career of alcoholics than had been thought. When the impairment is gross the patient may be incapacitated and have to stay permanently in hospital. Dementia is not an inevitable consequence of chronic alcoholism. The majority of chronic alcoholics who have been successfully treated are able to function without evidence of intellectual impairment. Once present, however, dementia is irreversible.

All the foregoing conditions are unquestionably organic in aetiology. They are caused by chemical or structural abnormalities in the brain. Other psychological conditions are found which have not been shown to have such an organic basis. These are called 'functional' disorders. This name puts them in line with the majority of psychoses unrelated to alcohol, which, indeed, they in some measure resemble: so much so that there is still controversy whether, when these conditions develop in an alcoholic, the drinking was their cause or merely the first symptom of them. Such doubts cannot be altogether resolved, and it is wiser just to describe the conditions than to attempt authoritative explanation.

The first of these is *pathological jealousy*. Generally affecting men, but sometimes women too, the jealousy is directed towards the spouse, who is believed to be unfaithful. Pathological jealousy goes far beyond normal jealousy, although it may at first involve no more than fleeting suspicions which can be easily resisted. Such ideas are commonly described by male alcoholics and, indeed, their wives may at first not be distressed by the observant attention which their husbands give them. As jealousy becomes more intense, the alcoholic may still retain the ability to doubt his suspicions, although these are now disturbing enough to feature as a symptom. In severe cases, belief in the spouse's infidelity reaches delusional force. It may not be overcome by reasoning, and resists clear-cut evidence which rebuts specific allegations. The jealous husband seizes upon any chance remark that his wife makes, any passing glance she may receive from a man, to feed his suspicions. He searches her handbag for letters and her underwear for tell-tale signs. The jealous wife looks for lipstick marks on his person or clothing. Protestations of innocence are not believed. The alcoholic frequently upbraids the spouse and alcoholic husbands all too often beat their wives either for their supposed adultery or to try to make them confess. Such a wife's lot may become unbearable, yet so limited is the field of her husband's delusions and so rational is he in every other particular that it is next to impossible to be sure where the truth lies and, if necessary, to order his compulsory detention in hospital. Needless to say, he will not go voluntarily. Separation is often the only practicable course, although its immediate effect is to fan the flame of suspicion. Divorce courts frequently hear testimony of pathological jealousy, and it may result in murder. One explanation for its occurrence in association with alcoholism is to be found in our theory of the *paranoid shift*, which we describe in Chapter 8 as one of the stages of alcoholism. Psychoanalysts maintain that pathological jealousy is a manifestation of disguised homosexuality. It is a defence for the patient against the recognition of his own inclinations and at the same time, covertly, a gratification of them. He projects on to his wife his own unrecognized feelings for the other man. This view is far from being shared by most psychiatrists.

Once pathological jealousy has reached the stage of delusions the outlook for recovery is not good. Some patients develop an illness resembling schizophrenia. However, less extreme forms of jealousy commonly fade if the patient gives up drinking. Morbid jealousy is more common among male than female alcoholics, but it does occur in women also, with the roles reversed. One of our patients, for instance, was delusionally convinced that her husband was having an affair with her best friend, but suddenly switched to an equally delusional belief that he was having a homosexual affair when she found a trace of faecal staining on his underpants. An alcoholic, through self-neglect, may indeed disaffect the partner.

Another psychotic condition is *alcoholic hallucinosis*. The patient, who is fully conscious, hears voices, characteristically very vivid, which commonly talk about him or her in obscene language. The hallucinations may clear up if drinking stops, but sometimes, even with abstinence, they continue for years. One patient, a bookmaker, described how he had been 'on the line' to such voices for ten years, during which time he had been able to continue working and drinking. When he gave it up they stopped, but the first time he relapsed they returned, and although he was subsequently able to remain teetotal they persisted permanently afterwards. Auditory hallucinations of this sort are quite different from the vivid, transient and disorganized hallucinations, usually visual, which occur with alcoholic tremulousness and delirium tremens.

I clearly heard a conversation between my mother and my domestic help, which I thought was taking place outside the kitchen. Throughout the day, I frequently asked members of the household to repeat what they had just said as I had not heard it properly, only to be told that no one had uttered a word. I frequently heard my husband's voice calling me, as if he were upstairs or in the hall.

The next day I was defrosting my refrigerator when I distinctly heard my husband in his office, which is completely away from our house. I heard him having consultations with three different people, then dictating letters and talking to his secretary. It seemed to me that I was actually hearing what was happening at that precise moment.

During the early afternoon I was most disturbed to hear a strange male voice which was loud and clear, and claimed to be my conscience. By this time I was in a state of agitation; I sincerely believed this to be my conscience rebuking me. I was getting absolutely no peace from this voice, which was accompanied by music, and a mixed choir all of which had the quality of what I would call Church music. After the evening meal was over this became so loud and persistent that I felt anyone in the room with me could not fail to hear it as well as I was receiving it. Therefore I escaped by myself on every possible occasion and even found myself talking aloud in reply to this 'conscience'. My husband became very curious as to the reason for my frequent disappearances and, in the end, I took him into my confidence. As the evening wore on, the nature of the voice and music changed completely and became almost raucous. The voice introduced himself as 'Jimmy Young' from Glasgow, my hometown. I have never at anytime in my life personally known anyone by this name. The tone of voice at times was very polished, but sometimes it assumed a very decided Glasgow accent. Gradually it became louder and louder, and almost mocking and jeering at me, to the extent that I became angry with myself for being so taken in as ever to believe this could be my conscience. I began to be convinced that this was some extraordinary type of radio wave which some cranks had been able to 'tune in' to me.

This patient recovered completely; unfortunately not all patients do.

There is no evidence to incriminate any organic process. The condition of alcoholic hallucinosis is not a withdrawal symptom, nor is it due to a vitamin deficiency: it is much more closely related to schizophrenia, and, if it persists, it cannot be distinguished from that disease except by the history. Fortunately it is not common.

Suicide

Many alcoholics kill themselves. The suicide rate for male alcoholics admitted for treatment in a London psychiatric hospital, for instance, was eighty-six times higher than that for men in the same age groups in the general London population; the rate for those who had been admitted to an observation ward was seventy-six times as high.[3] A Scandinavian study of 220 male alcoholics revealed that 7 per cent kill themselves during a five-year period after leaving hospital.[4] Alcoholics who commit suicide may well do so after losing their spouse or their job. Every doctor who is responsible either for alcoholics or for people who deliberately poison or injure themselves knows how commonly the two are found in combination. In Edinburgh, 44 per cent of all men admitted to hospital in 1986 having attempted suicide revealed a drinking problem, and 15 per cent of these had symptoms of alcoholism; 20 per cent of females similarly admitted had a drinking problem.[5] In 1986, 66 per cent of male admissions and 48 per cent of female admissions consumed alcohol prior to their attempted suicide. As long ago as 1900, reports were appearing showing that suicide rates were high in occupations where alcoholism was rife. In different countries at different periods close parallels have been shown between fluctuations in alcohol consumption and male mortality from suicide.

The importance of these findings cannot be too strongly stressed. They indicate three things. First, even the slightest intimation of suicidal intent by an alcoholic must be taken very seriously; second, a close watch must be kept upon all alcoholics before, during and after treatment, so that any suicidal intentions can be detected in time to prevent tragedies. Even so, some will not be preventable, because the suicidal impulse can arise very suddenly in association with intoxication. The clinical impression is that if the dependence is cured then the risk of suicide is very considerably reduced. Third, a history of alcoholism should be looked for in every person who deliberately takes an overdose.

Alcohol and Pregnancy

Over the last twenty years, and particularly in the United States, concern has been voiced about the risk to the foetus caused by maternal drinking during pregnancy. The 'foetal alcohol syndrome' has been described in which there is a distortion of the bones of the face, and sometimes other bodily lesions, together with a reduced intelligence in the infant which is continued into adult life.[6] Two things must at once be said: first, this syndrome is extremely rare, and second, the mothers of these babies had been drinking very great quantities of alcohol. Nowadays those who had earlier stressed the facial bone abnormality acknowledge the great rarity of this and are worried instead about the low birth weight of the children and a possible low intelligence. Since many heavily drinking women also smoke a great deal, have other social disabilities and may neglect themselves and avoid antenatal care, it has not proved easy to ascertain the part played by the drinking itself. However, a French study[7] of 9,000 births, which took account of the smoking factor, failed to show a single case of the foetal alcohol syndrome. Other physical abnormalities which were not severe occurred among the infants of heavy- and light-drinking mothers in about equal proportions. The mean birth weight of babies born to the heavier-drinking mothers was marginally less than the other babies. Intelligence was not rated as the babies were then too young.

The foetal brain is most vulnerable to factors which might inhibit its growth at about the eleventh week of pregnancy, when many mothers may not be aware that they are pregnant. Fortunately, many pregnant women feel even before they know of their pregnancy that they do not enjoy drinking; both the taste and the effects of alcohol displease them.[8] Thus the desirable cutting down of drinking occurs fortuitously, without it being undertaken by the mother for health reasons. Unfortunately, the women who persist in drinking tend to be heavy drinkers who, because of dependence, cannot stop. These are exactly the mothers who we should most strive to influence, but exhortation, without anti-alcoholism help, is unlikely to be successful.

What advice can we give? Obviously, if a pregnant woman does not drink there can be no risk of alcohol affecting the foetus. On the other hand, there is no evidence to convince us that occasional light social drinking during pregnancy will harm the baby, and mothers-to-be need therefore feel neither fearful nor guilty. Women who are continuous steady drinkers, or intermittent heavy drinkers, would be well advised to cut down for their own good, as well as for the sake of their child. To put the matter in perspective, smoking during pregnancy presents a graver risk to the child. If a woman is in doubt or worried, she should consult her doctor.

Chapter 4

Social Organization and Drinking

The study of different cultures sheds light on Western drinking. Anthropologists have frequently found that inferences can be drawn from pre-industrial cultures more readily than from post-industrial ones, but that their conclusions then prove relevant to more differentiated societies. Only where the culture fosters drinking will alcoholism be widespread. Whatever the individual's psychological difficulties may be, unless the social circumstances are appropriate he or she will deal with these in another way than by excessive drinking. This fact must be kept in mind when we come, in the next chapter, to cover the effect of personality. The cultural soil, so to speak, must be right for the seeds of an individual's alcoholism to develop.

Favourable cultural conditions for promoting alcoholism must obviously include availability of supplies. But this by itself is not enough. From a sociological standpoint, everybody can be regarded as potentially alcoholic; recourse to alcohol is a possible way, then, for an individual to relieve tension.

In simple cultures, everyone has their place, with an importance and a dignity that the group recognizes. As social differentiation increases in more advanced cultures, more rules are required. Those individuals who find themselves hard-pressed to fulfil the requirements imposed on them become anxious because they must suppress and inhibit some of their urges in order to conform.

From society's requirements rules emerge which check individual behaviour. As a society's rules become more complex, and especially where their enforcement is harsh and punitive, the individuals have to limit the extent to which they can act solely in accord with their own wishes. Restrictions tend to be most stringent where they relate to aggressive and sexual behaviour. The threat of retaliatory punishment evokes anxiety in a person whenever sexual or hostile urges are aroused. Because these are vigorous urges, a powerful conflict is set up in the individual.

Recourse to alcohol may be used, if the society permits, to facilitate release of these proscribed urges or to help the drinker to avoid situations that provoke them.

This is a use of drinking adopted to deal with tensions that the organization of society has imposed. On the other hand, in very simple cultures drinking consolidates group cohesiveness, and alcoholism is reported as rare. The emotions aroused by alcohol are shared in the group setting and enhanced by singing and ritual. Drunkenness, too, is a shared behaviour. It takes the form of periodic revels. These enable the individuals to experience and express their close links with each other. In such societies anxiety and fear are significant not only as individual experiences but also as group phenomena. Horton,[9] an anthropologist, recorded that the frequency with which drunkenness occurs in such societies is determined by the amount of anxiety and fear experienced by the group. In a study of 118 cultures in Africa, Asia and the Americas he was able to relate the frequency of drunkenness to two indices of social anxiety: first, insecurity about food supplies, and second, stresses from acculturation by contact with Western civilization which weakened social patterns and kinship ties. The more these factors operated, the more drunkenness there was.

The combination of group fears and the individuals' repressed urges becomes too great. Something has to give. These societies have evolved an adaptive pattern designed to relax their restraints from time to time. Popular festivities take place during which group drunkenness occurs. Sexual and aggressive behaviour at such times do not incur censure, and exposure, suggestive body movements, intercourse, arguments and brawls are permitted. Apart from these orgies, drunkenness is rare and alcoholism does not occur.

When the organization of society becomes still more differentiated, as in modern European society, acting-out behaviour of this sort is no longer tolerated, even on the rare occasions when group drinking is still permitted. On such public days of celebration, drunkenness is more excused than at other times, but excesses of aggressive and sexual behaviour are not condoned. The excessive drinker in Western societies drinks against his society. Excessive drinking becomes almost a rebellious gesture. The scene is now set, the conditions are right, for some people to become alcoholics.

In different Western nations, society has organized itself in diverse ways, and from country to country patterns both of drinking and of excessive drinking vary. Climate and geography, economics and local customs, all influence national patterns of drinking.

In France many people get all or part of their income from the production and sale of alcoholic drinks. These people are wholly or partly dependent on the wine and spirit industries for their livelihoods. In a quite literal sense they are supported by alcohol. It is understandable, therefore, that four fifths of French people believe that wine is 'good for one's health'. Indeed, when surveyed thirty years ago a quarter held that it was indispensable. Large quantities of alcohol are taken regularly by many Frenchmen, without them considering that they are drinking too much or that they are misusing alcohol. Men who were asked the question how much wine a working man could drink daily 'without any inconvenience' gave answers which averaged two litres. The consumption of large quantities of wine was thought quite proper by the people surveyed. French drinkers consume wine steadily throughout the day; these inveterate drinkers constantly have a high amount of alcohol in their bodies. They are chronically poisoned, although they rarely show very disturbed behaviour. Their drinking becomes a problem as much because of the insidious physical consequences as because of psychological or behavioural consequences. Indeed, French psychiatrists used to disagree among themselves whether alcoholism should be regarded as a psychiatric problem at all. Nowadays, however, they are persuaded (not so all French physicians) that it is.

Italy, too, has a considerable economic stake in alcohol production. More arable land is under viticulture than in France. Not only are alcoholism rates high in Italy but the death rate from cirrhosis is one of the highest in the world. It is interesting, however, that nowadays industrial workers, especially those who are single or separated, make up the majority of alcoholics.

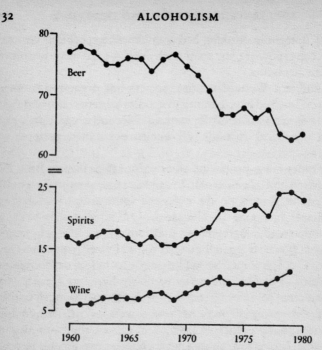

Figure 1 Type of drink: Approximate percentage of total consumption in UK

In Britain and North America, drinking takes a different pattern. It is not continuous throughout the day, nor is alcohol taken mainly with meals as a shared family activity. Furthermore, a large amount of spirits is drunk. Beer and spirits are the most prevalent drinks, in contrast to the wine of Continental countries. Moreover, drink is taken rapidly, either when work is finished or after the evening meal, to produce a sudden rise in the level of alcohol in the body. This method of drinking leads to drunkenness, which is the hallmark of British and American excessive drinking. While beer remains the dominant beverage in the United Kingdom, accounting for over half of all alcohol purchased, wine drinking has risen enormously and so has consumption of spirits (see Figure 1).

Five types of establishment are licensed to sell drink for consumption on the premises in Britain: hotels, restaurants, public houses, bars and registered clubs. Other places, off-licences and licensed grocers, are permitted to sell drink for consumption away from the premises.

Recently there has been a great rise, a four-fold increase over six years, in the granting of licences to grocery supermarkets that permit them to offer drink for sale. Moreover, the check-out counter system of such shops make it very difficult to prevent sales to people under age.

The pub is the principal locus of drinking in Britain. In England the public house provides drink in a pleasant and convivial social atmosphere; in many, music is part of the setting; games, darts, fruit machines and the like are available. In most pubs women are welcome, although this is not invariably the case. Publicans can easily create an atmosphere that is either acceptable to women or not. There is, for instance, the simple matter of the provision of toilets. Nevertheless, since most public houses are owned by brewing companies and these have been at pains to advertise to attract women, there has been a corresponding change in the facilities and ambiance provided. The old division into saloon and public bars is almost gone, in favour of open lounge accommodation, more suitable for drinking by the family. It is comparatively rare now to find public houses where women are treated as unwelcome, even if there are many where they may not choose to go unaccompanied.

Many people become very attached to their own pub so that they rarely go elsewhere to drink. Each pub thus develops a band of regulars who may strike up friendships and who, at the very least, feel at home in each other's company. One of the beneficent features occasioned by women in public houses is that these no longer seem to be, at least in the majority of instances, simply drinking shops in a one-sex setting. The effects of this upon personal behaviour and group conduct have been considerable. The old atmosphere was conducive to pathological drinking. The modern public house permits the influence of social conventions to restrain drunkenness and its consequent behaviours.

The pattern of drinking during the week varies with locality. Males in Scotland reported an average of 3·0 drinking days in the past week compared with 3·6 by men in England and Wales. The corresponding number of days in Northern Ireland was still lower, only 2·3. The trend among women was the same: an average of 2·7 drinking days in England and Wales; 2·1 in Scotland; and 1·6 in Northern Ireland.[10] These variations have been held to connote that in Scotland and Northern Ireland drunkenness is more common, since drinking is concentrated into fewer days.

The number of people engaged in the drink industry in Britain is considerable. At the start of the 1950s, Seebohm Rowntree and Lavers[11] made a conservative estimate of 340,000. This figure did not include those engaged in the wholesale distribution of alcoholic liquor. To give perspective to this total they pointed out that it was approximately 50 per cent more than the number of workers engaged in all sections of the gas, water and electricity supply industries. At present, approximately 750,000 people are employed in the production and distribution of alcoholic drinks in the United Kingdom, according to the Brewers Society. In 1978, three quarters of the adult population visited a public house at least once, and 12 per cent of men and 10 per cent of women visited a pub every day. More detailed information about British drinking is given in Chapter 13.

In the United States, alcoholism is rightly recognized as a very serious public health problem. Social concern about alcoholism is greater than in Britain. Yet on the other hand social attitudes towards drinking have been responsible for the magnitude of the problem. From its earliest Puritan days, organized American public opinion has never been able to come to terms with alcoholics, but has oscillated between severe condemnation and frankly vicarious admiration. In 1919 the United States introduced prohibition. The effect of this harsh measure remains a disputed matter, but there is little doubt that inability to enforce it, together with waning popular support, combined to make it fail. Equally strong public attitudes in the United States led to the formation both of the National Council on Alcoholism and of Alcoholics Anonymous.

The significance of religion in relation to drinking has been much studied, because of the low alcoholism rates among Jews,

Moslems and Mormons. (Higher rates occur in predominantly Roman Catholic countries, as we have observed.) Mormons will expel a member because of drinking, so it is especially interesting that among Mormon college students there is a high incidence of drinking to intoxication with socially harmful results. Their excessive drinking expresses a rebellion against cultural trends, religious pressures in particular. Methodists are brought up in constant awareness of the evil consequences of drinking. Total abstinence is enjoined upon their members. Yet during their student days they had more drinking problems than either Jews or Episcopalians. It was found that those students who drank generally concealed the fact from their fathers.[12] However, this key study has recently been analysed by Makela,[13] who took equal account of all the subjects, including those who did not use alcohol (whose significance the original investigation minimized). When he did so it emerged that social complications caused by drinking were more common among Episcopalians than Methodists. It cannot in fact be claimed, from the findings of this study, that abhorrence of drinking in the parental home during childhood increased the chance of abnormal drinking in later life.

Jews have a low prevalence of alcoholism. To explain this low rate, it is suggested that, whilst Jews have no taboos against the moderate use of alcoholic beverages, which indeed play an integral part in social and ceremonial activity, drinking to excess has always been sternly disapproved of. Because the outlet of normal social drinking is permitted and approved, Jews seeking to express their personal conflicts do not turn to excessive drinking.

Our review of drinking habits permits some generalization. When a society approves drinking and tolerates drunkenness, whether all the time or on special occasions, then many people will drink to excess. Because they will not be doing anything proscribed, they will not be acting antisocially, and they will feel no guilt. Consequently, psychological abnormalities will not frequently be found in the excessive drinkers. If, however, the society disapproves of drinking, it will be especially critical of those who drink to excess. The population of excessive drinkers will then consist mainly of two groups: those who seek to rebel against the social group, and those whose inner tensions are so great that they must obtain the relief afforded by alcohol, regardless of society's censure. Excessive drinkers in such societies are judged by their fellows to be morally weak and self-indulgent. Being products of their society they share this estimate of themselves. Hence they experience much guilt. The condemnation by society and their own sense of shame conspires to bring about their isolation.

Historical Changes in Drinking Habits

Throughout history, the pattern of drinking in Britain has changed with modifications made in the organization of society. Of the days of Queen Anne, Trevelyan[14] writes:

> Drunkenness was the acknowledged national vice of Englishmen of all classes, though women were not accused of it. A movement for total abstinence was out of the question, in days before tea or coffee could be obtained in every home and when the supply of drinking water was often impure. But tracts in favour of temperate drinking were freely circulated by religious bodies and anxious patriots, setting forth with attractive detail the various and dreadful fates of drunkards, some killed attempting to ride home at night, others seized by a fit while blaspheming, all gone straight to Hell. Among the common folk, ale still reigned supreme; but ale had a new rival worse than itself in the deadly attraction of bad spirits. The acme of cheap spirit-drinking was not indeed reached till the reign of George II, in the days of Hogarth's 'Gin Lane', but things were already moving in that direction.
>
> Meanwhile the upper classes got drunk sometimes on ale and sometimes on wine. It is hard to say whether the men of fashion or rural gentry were the worst soakers. But perhaps the outdoor exercise taken by the fox-hunting, sporting, and farming squire made him better able to absorb his nightly quantum of October, than the gamester and politician of St James's Square to escape the ill effects of endless Whig toasts in port and Tory toasts in French claret and champagne. Magistrates often appeared on the bench heated with wine; courts martial, by a prudent provision of the Mutiny Act, might only take place before dinner.

The worst excesses of the gin-palace era of cheap spirits were checked in 1751 by an Act which taxed them highly and stopped their retail sale by distillers and shopkeepers. Even after this, however, as many as an eighth of the deaths of London adults were attributed by medical men to an excess of spirit-drinking. Tea became a strong competitor to alcohol toward the end of the eighteenth century, but the industrial revolution brought with it a resurgence of excessive drinking, particularly in the cities. Alcohol became for many the only recourse from the miseries inflicted by direst poverty. In the wake of this orgy of mass drinking the temperance movement grew up in the latter half of the nineteenth century. Doctors, clergymen and others not only urged the merits and indeed duties of temperance upon a largely heedless public but, more to the point, succeeded in producing in 1914 effective legislation licensing the places which could sell drink and fixing hours for its purchase and consumption. Trevelyan comments:

> When Queen Victoria died, drinking was still a great evil from the top to the bottom of society, more widely prevalent than in our day, but decidedly less than when she came to the throne.[15]

These laws abated some of the worst excesses, at a time when some of the widespread social misery was being reduced. The beneficial impact of the improved licensing laws was rapidly felt, but the advantages of temperance were much slower to be appreciated. It was not until during and after the First World War that drunken behaviour began to be considered unacceptable in every walk of society. During the depression, in the late twenties and early thirties, there was once again an increase in drunkenness, which for a long time had moved in step with unemployment. However, gross public drunkenness, people lying paralytic in the streets, is now a rare sight in Britain.

In the 1950s a new phenomenon began to be apparent in Britain: young teenage drunkenness, probably as a consequence of the increased affluence of this age group. The increase both in drunkenness and in alcoholism in the young is rightly causing serious concern.

Chapter 5

Personality Factors in Alcoholics

Personality is complex. A part of it changes from day to day, with alterations in mood and as a response to events or to people; such variations are evanescent. A more enduring part of the personality is made up of beliefs and attitudes which are not readily alterable; this is the side of people that others describe when discussing them, and which they know as themselves. This more enduring part of personality is capable only of very slow change as the person takes on new responsibilities or undergoes great emotional experiences. An even deeper part of the personality contains the drives and motivations which give the self its impetus. Many psychologists consider this core to be all but immutable.

To an observer, an individual's personality is manifested by behaviour; it consists of the total of his or her characteristic actions and reactions. Abnormality of personality consists of an excess or a lack of a number of attributes, such as assertiveness, common to us all.

Intuitive appraisals of personality, such as we all make when summing people up, are very different from scientific assessments. In day-to-day life our own feelings enter into our judgements of personality. Psychologists aim to eliminate this subjective element. They may do so by isolating particular traits of personality, such as sociability or aggression, and measuring their degree in different people. Or they may consider the total personality of those people they study and attempt a systematic classification of them into recognized stereotypes.

We can study the personality of alcoholic patients but we cannot say how much our findings are applicable to all alcoholics, since it is only a minority that are examined by a psychiatrist or psychologist. There is no single alcoholic personality. Nevertheless, psychiatrists dealing with alcoholics recognize characteristic types which occur frequently, either alone or in combination, and it is these which we shall now describe.

The Personality of the Alcoholic

The effects of alcohol have already been set out. The question arises: why do people drink, knowing what the effect will be?

On one hand, as we have seen, people drink because it is the custom. Much attention has been paid to another reason for drinking. This focuses on the fact that the social drawbacks and self-doubt of many people can be relieved by drinking. People who need Dutch courage find that they are indeed made bolder by drink. We need to understand the origins of poor self-esteem in certain people in order to grasp why some turn to alcohol as a means for gaining, albeit transiently, confidence and assertiveness. A person terrified of appearing feeble and inefficient when entertaining callers, a worker afraid of his or her senior, someone fearful of not responding adequately in sexual intercourse, and any diffident person in consternation prior to a public appearance: such people discover that drinking can allay terrors, confer calm and dispel dread. Unfortunately, as time passes, an increasing amount of alcohol, rising progressively to a degree that can disorganize the personality, is needed to reduce timidity, inadequacy, lack of confidence and a sense of inferiority.

These are social terrors. We need also to explain why some people drink when on their own. Drinking can change the inner state of a person. Alcohol is psychotropic. It sets up a feeling tone of pleasure, tranquillity or even elation. 'I reach the ceiling of my world,' one man explained. Alcoholics in treatment are sometimes encouraged to paint, and quite regularly the picture resulting is of a ship, occasionally with the caption: 'Sailing Away'. A person can regularly arrive at euphoria simply through drinking; a drinking session (often without the demands of associating with other people) can confer chemical hedonism, almost effortless contentment. Obtaining this change of one's inner state is often the reason for drinking.

As a rough general statement, two sorts of personality can be singled out as prone to excessive drinking. People with the first lack self-confidence, have little self-esteem, and may even be disgusted with themselves. Often such people will have been deprived of affection in childhood, sometimes frankly neglected, or even mistreated. Women may describe cold, unloving mothers who expected the worst of them, or stepfathers who never regarded them affectionately; men may have been physically assaulted by parents, or as children made to feel wicked or depraved. 'Self-punitiveness' is a characteristic of such alcoholics as these, apparently long pre-dating the onset of alcoholism: for them alcohol brings respite from a pervading sense of insufficiency and inferiority and from constantly upbraiding themselves.

By contrast a second, very different type of person is quite free of self-loathing and not troubled in personal relations: such is the self-indulgent individual, who often was pampered in childhood by doting or anxious parents. The only son, perhaps younger than his sisters; the youngster for whom everything was done and on whom few demands were imposed, the sheltered beings who never really needed to fend for themselves. Such people can find that the harsh realities of work, personal relations and marriage add up to a bleak vista of obligations and responsibilities. These may be met more or less effectively, but there may also be the discovery that drinking can confer episodes of mental vacation. More than that, when under the influence of alcohol to the right extent, day-dreams or happy, perhaps exciting, reveries can be summoned to transform mundane existence.

In treatment, such hedonistic alcoholics bent on seeking euphoria through drink seem to do rather better than the self-punitive alcoholics who let up on themselves only when drinking. That aside, these two types of alcoholic indicate how differently the personality can be organized in pre-alcoholism: in some the discovery is that alcohol helps to reduce personal unease, while others come to depend on alcohol to confer a desired mental state of heightened contentment.

Related Personality Problems

One view of personality is that separate systems exist in the self, at different levels of awareness. Parts of the self are not accessible; these unrecognized parts can be wholly repugnant to the conscious self and, for this reason, are sometimes spoken of as 'ego-alien'. The disorder in the self which leads the person to morbid dependency on the drug will often not be at all clearly apparent to him or her. Indeed, people do not care to, or cannot, recognize these parts of themselves, since it is the embittered, enraged, resentful or defiant parts of the self which get suppressed because they are odious to the person.

When alcoholics overcome the dependence and stop drinking, the harmful effects of prolonged intoxication will be reversed, but they may still suffer from the effects of associated personality difficulties. These will be manifested especially as difficulties in relationships with other people.

Personality Disorders

We assess personality by observing how a person behaves and how he responds to the various events occurring in his or her life. In clinical terms personality is diagnosed by study of a person's traits (dependency and passivity, levels of hostility, degrees of pessimism, etc.), and by studying the person's relations with the important people in his or her life. If these are reasonably sustaining, coherent and emotionally rewarding, we judge the personality as normal. The personality is diagnosed as abnormal when the person's relations with other people are disturbed. They may be too dependent and clinging, unusually assertive and domineering, or too detached from people and unable to relate to them with ordinary warmth and responsiveness.

Personality can be disordered to varying degrees. Mild disorders may not be evident to anyone else, only apparent when people themselves disclose that they have social problems.

The most severe form of personality disorder is known as sociopathy (or psychopathy). Sociopaths cannot meet the rules or expectations of their social group. They live for the day and do not plan for the future. They are lacking in ordinary feelings and may be incapable of forming warm relationships, hence the term 'affectionless'. Antisocial sociopaths may be without a sense of guilt while perpetrating their mischief or crime, and without remorse subsequently. Aggressive sociopaths do serious harm to others, and can be violent: the coldness and callousness of such people are often extreme. Passive sociopaths sometimes become hoboes or aimless drifters if they don't have a tolerant family circle able to provide shelter despite the person's ineptitude at fending for himself or herself. It does not need clinical expertise to recognize sociopathy: these destructive or feckless people are well known in their social circles and neighbourhoods.

Personality and Alcoholism

Two separate matters call for consideration: the psychological attributes of the alcoholic which can help to cause alcoholism, and the effects which prolonged, continuous drinking exert on the personality. Traits or features sometimes viewed as characteristic of alcoholics may in fact also be the result of prolonged excessive drinking.

There is an important corollary to this. It is of course perfectly possible, indeed probable, that a latent, disguised aspect of personality, part of the 'unconscious mind', can be a part cause of excessive drinking, and only become apparent as actual observed behaviour when the alcoholic is drinking. Homosexual behaviour or criminal activity is an example. For this reason, after exploring personality traits preceding alcoholism, we go on to pay attention to personality features associated with alcoholics.

Nearly everybody drinks small amounts of alcohol when relating socially to other people, in pubs, at parties and at home. Alcohol certainly reduces inhibitions and thus can relieve social tension. Drinking alcohol makes people less shy and, equally useful socially, they usually get a little elated when they drink.

Studies conducted as drink takes effect on people have shown that alcohol increases the person's sense of power. Another finding from psychological research is that feelings of wanting to be taken care of, and to have dependency needs met, are at the basis of the satisfaction derived from drinking alcohol. Some investigators have therefore viewed alcoholics as dependent on others, not adequately free from their emotional tie with their mothers, excessively self-centred and incapable of being contented on their own.

Alcoholics can also be unduly self-indulgent. When they are disappointed or deprived of the satisfactions they seek, intense rage often arises – about which they feel guilty and for which they reproach and even punish themselves. This reverberating cycle of complicated feelings can be influenced by drinking, which increases their sense of self-esteem: the alcohol produces a sense of satisfaction, and also reduces rage and vengefulness, a relief to be welcomed because the sense of anger is subjectively painful. Further, drinking can punish those nearest to an alcoholic whom he or she sees as neglectful and insufficiently solicitous and responsive.

In general, therefore, such an alcoholic's personality will be marked by traits of passivity. A basically dependent person, when drinking, can become actually passive, without recognizing or owning up to this lapse into inactivity and irresponsibility. But this irresponsibility is then complicated by the other aspect of alcoholism, that alcoholics dare not reveal this passivity in ordinary social life and at work.

The Alcoholic's Independence

The basic passivity we have described therefore becomes masked by a determined and exaggerated forcefulness, which is not altogether convincing, and by a surface firmness and apparent independence. Some men can be seen very clearly as 'hung up' by a conflict between an urge to be blatantly masculine on the one hand, and a more submerged longing for 'passive gratification' on the other. Under the influence of alcohol, the alcoholic aspires to appear confident, secure and assertive. More than this, an effect of alcohol is actually to allow aggressive behaviour, without alcoholics having to acknowledge fully, when subsequently they become sober, how hostile they had been and hence suffering a dismaying recollection in an agony of guilt and contrition.

The family constellation of future alcoholics is of great relevance and interest. Here is a family background commonly found: a boy with a close emotional bond to a strong mother but with a weak father, consequently identifying psychologically with his mother and failing to do so with his father. He endorses and adopts his mother's designs for him, and repudiates or scorns the influence which his father, however weakly, could contribute. Our future alcoholic may in consequence have a social self which is his mother's creation, and he develops a basic feeling of weakness. He may subsequently over-correct his early feminine identification by a show of masculine bravado. Determined, rather indiscriminate sociability is both a means of telling the world that one is not weak, and at the same time of belonging socially to a social group that can persuade the alcoholic that he counts for something. Such a man may marry a strong wife, to recreate a similar influence to that which his mother had afforded, and also in the hope, which may be unconscious, of being sustained by a competent, effective spouse. When dominated in his marriage, the alcoholic can subdue his rage at being placed in the submissive position, reflecting as it may do his earlier dependence on his mother, by drinking.

Alcoholics, of course, do not themselves usually comprehend such explanations, but they can be useful to trained helpers because they convey an understanding of how a person's drinking career may have developed. They will also guide the course of inquiry needed to disclose the formative influences during youth and the alcoholic's private thoughts.

We have reviewed what personality is: the patterned cluster of traits or characteristics of the person. Many researchers have concluded that dependency needs and desires must be regarded as the most important psychological attributes of alcoholics, however adeptly disguised. This perspective orients the trusted adviser in his or her own behaviour towards the alcoholic. The personality of the alcoholic commonly revolves around the wish to be dependent and the compromises which alcoholics must develop to cope with conflicts over giving in to this longing. Their fear is that open expression of dependency will lose them their self-respect and, for a man, sense of masculinity; in a woman alcoholic a similar set of childhood events can give rise to her recognizing herself as weak in her adoption of a culturally acceptable female stance. Some alcoholics are indeed passive, blatantly meek and docile beings who rely on others, but many alcoholics strive to dispel all evidence of dependency on other people. Unfortunately, successful compromise usually eludes alcoholics, and the majority oscillate between their inner longings to be dependent and an outward bravado intended to give the appearance of independence.

Alcoholics are frequently hostile people, whether they show it or not, and aggressive impulses like dependent needs come to the surface. This is a dreadful aspect of alcoholism. Gentle people can be transformed, and often become enraged when drunk. Alcoholics may resort disastrously to violence. Or they can turn their anger against themselves and become depressed. Alcoholics may loathe themselves and describe themselves in terms of the utmost worthlessness and contempt. Anger (and depression, its counterpart when turned against the self) is profoundly disturbing in alcoholics as in other people, and the alcoholic relies heavily for self-protection on the mental deception known by the technical term of *denial*, that is, the refusal to recognize a glaring fact about oneself. Criticisms of work performance, for example, will not be acknowledged as a deterioration of skill caused by drink and attendant hangovers but will be ascribed by rationalization to such self-saving notions as the malice of a colleague. This represents the paranoid shift stage that we describe in Chapter 8. Adverse judgements are all the more intolerable because of the self-preservative over-evaluation often seen in alcoholics, amounting sometimes to self-aggrandizement. Such apparent superiority often masks a very considerable sense of inferiority, and an appalling dread of being despised and shunned.

The form of alcoholics' relations with others, and their general sociability, has been characterized as self-centred, short-term, exhibitionistic and more excessive than the occasion warrants, instead of being directed towards long-term social relations in which obligations are perceived and met. This does not do justice to other qualities which may as often be found among alcoholics. They can be sensitive, emotional, sympathetic and generous, outgoing people who like to be with others, although frequently the sincerity of their emotional ties to others may appear trivialized by their joviality, particularly when drinking. Investigators have identified some alcoholics as 'schizoid': such people are character-ized on the one hand by superficial, inconsistent and self-centred participation in inter-personal relationships and on the other by being basically isolated and wrapped up in their own interests and concerns.

Drinking leads to impulsiveness and irresponsibility, both of these being attributes liable to increase the social and personal vulnerability of the alcoholic. Outraged indignation, mawkish excuses to explain unmet obligations and ingratiating appeals for special consideration are off-putting even to those who want to give encouragement and support. As even closest associates turn away, disappointed, puzzled or disgusted, increased drinking comes tragically to serve as the only dependable way to counter the terrors of rejection and isolation.

The Personality in Established Alcoholism

For alcoholics, each day can be full of defeats. This may be because they drink particularly at times when demands are placed on them, with the result that they impair their abilities and do not meet expectations. The shame and disappointment of a failure in performance can then be reduced by further drinking. The only drawback is that performance is thus further impaired. In a face-to-face encounter, on the telephone, or even in a written com-munication, alcoholics' marred perceptions and responses are evi-dent to themselves, while they hope that the loss of mental agility, the slightly slurred speech, even the smell of alcohol, may not be noticed. Some alcoholics on the contrary remain sober for special duties or challenges, when they are socially visible, and drink with relief once the task is accomplished. Alcoholics are vulnerable in two ways. First, they have personal drives and impulses, some-times masked, which clearly impose tensions and stresses. Second, equal attention should be given to their problems in relation to other people and the strained relationships, sometimes with the opposite sex, that give rise to the urge to drink.

This account of personality development, and the particular forms that the development may take in alcoholics, allows us now to look in detail at the personality types that we find in alcoholic patients. We shall concentrate especially on the types met with in alcoholics who have not reached the stage of mental deterioration, as this itself distorts personality.

Before embarking on the descriptions, however, we must observe that many alcoholics do not fit closely into any of these types, just as many whose personality development has been different from what we have outlined may turn into alcoholics. Nevertheless, just as we have described the predominant developmental features, we now portray the commonest personalities to be found amongst alcoholics. Anyone who sees a lot of alcoholics will undoubtedly come across each of these typologies many times.

Personality Patterns of Established Alcoholics

The Immature Personality

Some people do not reach the level of emotional development appropriate to adulthood. Arrested development of an aspect of personality at any stage leads to immaturity of personality. Some adults, for instance, cannot detach themselves from their parents' home. Others are extremely self-centred, unable to feel tenderness towards anyone else; such people cannot form an intimate and stable relationship with another person. Still others have a child-like need for approval and admiration. There are others who show great promise at school but who subsequently fail to realize what had been hoped for them and what they had hoped for themselves. Such people are preoccupied with private nostalgic memories of what might have been, boasting about those few things they have actually accomplished. It is a characteristic of all these immature people that in spite of their obvious assets they live unproductively.

We have described the unduly close relationship that many alcoholics have had with their mothers. One woman patient got drunk and suddenly burst out: 'There is a heaven and we will be together again, mother — oh, how I want to die!' Such intense and persistent ties to the mother are more characteristic of male alcoholics and may remain prominent even when the alcoholism is in remission. A forty-seven-year-old man, extremely cooperative in treatment, said in great distress that he had to confess that he had been deceiving the doctors for weeks; although he was not sure he was right to do so he wanted to correct the information he had given, namely that his mother had died of cancer. In fact she died of drink. This was the first time he had brought himself to disclose her 'lapse'; he had never even told his wife.

> I thought it unfair to her memory. But after a lot of thought, as the days passed, I thought I should tell the truth about her. I sincerely apologize, but I could not help myself. There were ten children before me in our family, and one after. I was nobody, but I got a lot of pleasure out of doing little things for my mother. When the children had all gone to bed she would sit by the fire, I would get out of bed and brush and comb her lovely long black hair for an hour. There must have been something soothing in this, as she thought it made her sleep better.

No other relationship that he had experienced in his life had been of such intensity.

The attachment to the mother can be still more extreme, a passion which can engulf the son so extravagantly that his life is entirely distorted by the prolonged dependence. A man who had had a few drinks before a group-treatment session and was therefore less guarded than usual, told his fellow alcoholics that he used always to drop in for a cup of coffee at his mother's house each morning on the way to work. He then burst out that he hated his father. When he was five he had seen his father slap his mother's face. That had spoilt his life. He had 'toddled' from the house into a field, vowing never to forgive his father, and he never had done so. That was why he drank: he would get himself drunk and then go to his parents' home expressly to rouse his father by his intoxicated state. It gratified him to make his father distressed and angry. 'Can you wonder I am still single?' he demanded. The other members tried to divert the conversation, but he would have none of it. When he was a little lad, he said, at the time of the slap, he had vowed he would wait for his father to die and then look after his mother himself. The others exclaimed with surprise, but he repeated that he would never marry; instead he would devote himself to his mother.

Adults who have their energies bound up in obsolete relationships are only partially susceptible to the influence of current experiences. They are bent on living out in the present a family myth which they conceived in childhood. Because the myth is personal and kept secret it cannot be influenced and corrected by real events. Dependent adults who cling because of an inner, private logic, to an outworn parental relationship, often sustained in fantasy long after the parent is dead, suffer serious limitations in their present life and cannot undertake the roles which experiences in adulthood create for them. These sorts of people turn to drink because their unreal fantasies of a golden relationship with a parent provide such a satisfying and nourishing world for them that the real world has nothing to offer of comparable value. When actual situations conflict with their fantasies they drink so as not to be aware of them. They escape into a world where reality does not penetrate. We have described their recourse to drink as though it were both conscious and deliberate, but this is not usually so. The fantasy world may perhaps be present only as a vague feeling-state. Drinking lessens the tension of conflict by permitting fantasy to predominate over a subdued reality.

The Self-indulgent Personality

Children need help, protection and affection while they are growing up, but each of these can be overdone. When children find tasks they have set themselves too difficult they ought to be helped, but there are some parents who rush in with assistance before the child's own resources and imagination have been employed. Children of over-protective parents, deprived of the satisfaction of discovery and personal achievement, get alternative gratifications by insisting that everything be done for them as if they were still infants. They fail to develop self-confidence or learn self-reliance. Children need to be guarded from common dangers, but some parents shield them from all possible hurt so that there is a scarcely a thing they are allowed to do on their own if the parents can imagine the smallest risk. They want to obviate discomfort of any sort; in case the child might be unhappy they will not leave him or her with other children of their own age. As a result the child becomes fearful of separation from his or her parents and never learns the social skills needed to mix easily with, be accepted by, and enjoy the company of peers. He or she will remain socially clumsy.

Such people remain self-indulgent in adult life. They are unable to accept frustrations. They live for, expect, and must have, easy and continuous gratification. To be thwarted is intolerably painful. They often eat a lot, chew sweets and smoke. All these activities have been viewed as expressions of a persisting infantile urge to find satisfactions akin to sucking. Drinking serves a similar end. Certainly there are alcoholics who actively enjoy the sensation of drinking. Those who suppose that alcohol dependence is all misery are wrong. A journalist spoke of 'my long love affair with drink'. For these alcoholics, to drink is a celebration. They are sybarites, isolating the pleasurable parts of reality. When drinking they dim the lights, play music and even at times costume themselves. They are expansive and boastful: 'When I drink I become an admiral.' They strive for super-pleasure. Yet self-indulgence deprives them of self-control; regulation of behaviour becomes increasingly difficult to achieve. The joys derived from a drink are a synthetic gratification which the alcoholic knows were not earned. Perhaps this is why there is often a tinge of disappointment in their description: 'I get to the top of my world, but usually it wasn't what I really wanted.'

The self-indulgent alcoholic, therefore, drinks for two reasons. It reduces the personal discomforts which arise whenever wishes are frustrated, and it provides a gratification that is always available and dependable. Of all alcoholics, the self-indulgent is most likely to drift into alcoholism without realizing it, and to take to drink like a voluptuary.

The Person with Sexual Problems

People who are not well-adjusted sexually fall into three categories. Some have little sexual drive; they are unlikely to become alcoholic unless they marry someone who interprets their apparent indifference as a personal slight. In that case they may turn to drink in an attempt to increase ardour or to escape from their spouses' or their own recriminations.

The second group of alcoholics with sexual problems are those whose sexual drives, though normally directed, cannot be realized because they have a fear of all dealings with the opposite sex. They may blush and feel uncomfortable in their presence; they find it difficult to carry on casual conversation and are daunted by the possibility of physical contact and petrified by the idea of intercourse. Some of these individuals express quite unreal notions about sexual activity. They may confide to the doctor ideas that sex is objectionable and that intercourse is unclean and leads to disease; or else they may romanticize sexual relations, maintaining that any physical contact sullies their purity. Another common rationalization is that intercourse is physically weakening. All these are unconscious devices hiding more basic fears of being harmed by intercourse or of proving impotent. Impotence is common among alcoholics, some of whom say they overcome it with drink. Certainly it may antedate the onset of drinking. A railwayman found that when he tried to have intercourse at sixteen he was unable to have an erection. He became engaged at twenty-four but would not marry because after months of trying he remained impotent. Twelve years later he was still single and, now alcoholic, regarded his almost nightly masturbation as a type of sedative.

The third category comprises the sexual deviants. For them either the object of love is not a person of the opposite sex (we refer principally to homosexuals), or a person of the opposite sex is the love object but normal intercourse does not provide the sexual satisfaction. Sadists, fetishists, and voyeurs come under this heading. After many interviews an alcoholic said:

> Oh, there's no actual perversion, not to my knowledge. It's just that I have standards, a sort of sexual 'must'. I'm not satisfied unless they are met. They are necessary for me to have an erection. The main point is the short skirt and high heels. Also a small waist, being generally of slight build and dieting to that end; the use of make-up, eyebrow shaping, jewellery – no woollen underwear or anything like that. There's some suffering involved as well. The shoe that's difficult to walk in, too tight. The fact that the person may be cold by not wearing warm underwear. The imposition of dieting, going hungry to lose weight. I won't have an erection because these things are carried out, but if they're not there I'm dissatisfied. I say to my wife to wear terylene for underwear, to get a new foundation and diet more. For a time she wore size 5 shoes when she should buy 5½. Now she has refused everything. She feels she's made a chattel. She says she'll come back to me only if there are no fetishes.

Sexual deviants take alcohol either in the hope that drinking will help them to achieve satisfactory normal behaviour, or to relieve the shame many feel concerning their perverse practices.

Homosexuals are in a special case. It is always possible to find a gay pub or a pub where drinking is still a male preserve. The homosexual enters the company of drinkers expressly to meet other homosexuals among them. In fact the exclusively male company and the disinhibiting factor of alcohol may temporarily bring out homosexual behaviour (not necessarily intercourse) in men who outside these circumstances are heterosexually oriented. Heterosexual men have sometimes awoken following a night's drinking to find themselves in bed with another man. These are people with a homosexual component to their personalities of which they may be unaware. A man may so strenuously repress the homosexual side of himself that he is excessively denigratory of homosexuals. A gentle and kindly alcoholic whose repressed homosexual qualities had long been apparent to his psychiatrist reported, 'I caught two Greeks having homosexual relations in the Army and I was successful in having them arrested.' A young divorced boilerman of a similar type said, 'I nearly killed a queer one day for trying something – I wrecked his flat.' Such a man after a number of psychiatric interviews sometimes confides that when uninhibited through drink he has responded to a homosexual approach. Others may suspect their ambivalent position in spite of their expression of distaste for homosexuals.

The Self-punitive Personality

It is normal to have aggressive feelings when conditions warrant. In the family, children are gradually trained to express reactions of anger with a moderation making it socially acceptable. If parents encourage their children to over-suppress hostile feelings while they are growing up it can lead to a fear of expressing anger in adult life. The outwardly docile products of such upbringing, even though they possess the intellectual and personality endowments to advance themselves, may be exploited by more dominating colleagues at work or may be disparaged by a relative or upbraided by a spouse without being able to respond with open anger to the provocations. The man who has to repress anger may at length be driven, by prolonged harsh treatment, to protest, but he will castigate himself afterwards, overcome by anxiety that drastic retaliation might follow his spell of self-assertiveness. For the most part he subdues his aggression and seeks to relieve the resultant discomfort. For him alcohol offers a method of doing so.

It is frequently chosen. The unassertive person we have described is aggressive when drunk; the hostile impulses, habitually concealed under normal social conditions, are released by the disinhibiting effect of alcohol, but that is not the reason for drinking: it is to relieve inner tension. Before this peace is achieved there is a stage in drinking when social controls are diminished, when intoxication dispels the timidity and caution which customarily confine the person. The transformation can be astonishing. While in this state they will vilify, rail, strike and destroy. They are usually aghast at themselves next morning, when they wake to a spouse's disapproval and see the damage they have done.

These four personality profiles will be recognized by all who come into contact with alcoholics either professionally or as companions. However, some alcoholics do not belong to any of these types. There are other people who drink excessively if they are emotionally overtaxed and cannot resolve the stressful situation by rational thinking. When a person can see only one element in a conflict, the other element being outside his or her awareness, no effort of will can solve the difficulty. This is the model for the development of neurosis, and if the person did not turn to drink a full-blown neurotic illness might have become manifest. In this sense, alcoholism may be seen to represent an attempt to ward off a psychological illness.

A company director drank whenever he was required to speak up for himself. If he had to make a proposal at a board meeting, or if he had to converse with a comparative stranger at a dinner, he would experience anxiety as a vague pain in the stomach: 'Like a bath running away' is how he described it. 'At dinner parties I'm absolutely hammering at myself to get a flicker out, to think of something, but I just can't.' At work, when called to exert his authority and correct an employee, he was stifled by the disproportionate rage he feared he might express. 'It's a curious thing to say, but I see red. My head gets bigger. I really do think I see red. I feel as if I might fall down. It distresses me that my position calls on me sometimes to hound people, to keep them up to the mark.' He was excessively strict with himself and felt it wrong to do things just for pleasure. So harshly did he judge himself that he was angry if he overslept by five minutes. He regarded his alcoholism as due to weak will.

That man was troubled by morbid unconscious fantasies. In some cases stresses arise out of actual events which are taxing beyond what anyone might be expected to bear. A patient who had been a war-time pilot told this story:

I had a horror of alcohol. I didn't touch it until I got my wings. Then three of my friends were killed in the space of three days. The expectation of life seemed to me six weeks, so I decided to try drinking. I started to take a couple of whiskies in the evening. Within eight months I found that I could drink whisky as fast as my companions in the squadron drank beer. I had quite a capacity. Throughout my service years I took a fair bucket.

He drank not only through fear but also with the thought that he should live as fully as he could in the few weeks of life remaining to him. For him alcohol heightened the joy of surviving each flying mission.

Drink is used as a medicine by people under stress. It does not serve as a tonic or as a sedative but as a pain-killer. With its help they can, temporarily at least, cope with their ordeals. Afterwards, when the stress is over, a man may get himself really drunk, this time to relax and unwind.

The categories of alcoholic personalities which we have described are not mutually exclusive. Many alcoholics share characteristics of more than one type. Moreover, they are not the only types of personality seen among excessive drinkers; no personality is immune from alcoholism and any person who sees a great deal of the problem knows of alcoholics who do not conform to these descriptions. Nevertheless, they are the commonest personalities to be met, and we have tried to indicate the function that alcohol serves for each of them. To sum these up, we see that the psychological satisfactions of drinking are:

(i) lessening of frustration with increase in gratification;
(ii) temporary attainment of a firmer social footing;
(iii) release from social inhibition of important parts of the self which normally have to be kept repressed at great cost to the individual's self-integration.

People with any of the personality types we have described do not necessarily become alcoholics or even drink to excess. In fact it is a minority who do. Drinking is only one possible recourse that they may adopt in order to come to terms with themselves or with others. These personality traits are common, and though possession of them may prevent individuals from living their lives as productively as they might otherwise do, they are not incompatible with a useful and ordered life.

We have described the personality types commonly found

among established alcoholics and the function that alcohol serves for each of them. Psychiatrists cannot say with any certainty how much these personality types are the product and how much the cause of drinking. They dare not presume that the facets of personality which they observe were there before excessive drinking began, for they know that the patient has inevitably been altered by the effects of drinking, not only physically but also psychologically and in his or her relationship with others. Long-term studies of individuals who become alcoholic have shown that psychological disorder is often a consequence of chronic intoxication.[16]

Chapter 6

The Causes of Alcoholism

Over the centuries four views have at various times held sway to account for alcoholism. These have been that it is a hereditary trait – coming from bad stock; that it arises from depravity of temperament; that it occurs when someone faced with life stresses that are too difficult to cope with seeks a helpful device – the bottle; or that it comes about simply as a result of the amount of alcohol drunk. Of these theories, that of depravity is no longer seriously put forward, although in popular culture the view of the alcoholic as a degenerate person persists. Hereditary principles began to be properly understood in this century, so that the earlier crude notion of alcoholism as inherited degeneracy is not now canvassed. Instead there is proper examination of possible hereditary features and we shall discuss these later. The third theory, that drinking is a device that some people seek to help them with their social predicaments held absolute sway in informed medical circles until very recently. It leads to the delineation of a classical triad of cause, well known to all students of medicine: that of the host, the environment and the agent. Alcohol is the agent. Someone, the host, who is faced by a life situation that is very difficult to deal with adopts a device to make things easier.

Sometimes the device of drinking is adopted to help surmount and overcome the problem; sometimes it is used to enable the person to avoid or escape it. Alcoholics do one or the other. In the long run they find that the device does not pay.

We shall return to the fourth theory, that alcoholism arises from alcohol itself, shortly. For the moment we need to explore further the man–problem–device model. This has two advantages for understanding alcoholism. First, it enables those who work with alcoholics to understand what is amiss with any particular sufferer; second, as we shall see, it directs attention to the three arms of treatment:

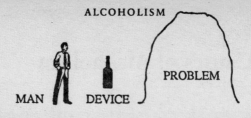

MAN   DEVICE   PROBLEM

Figure 2

(i) dealing with the person concerned, by offering support and sometimes by helping him or her to alter and strengthen the personality through psychological treatment or psychotherapy;

(ii) lessening the social predicament which is affecting the person;

(iii) eliminating the device by withdrawing the patient from alcohol and overcoming the dependence.

In practice, attention to each of these three matters is generally necessary for the successful treatment of every alcoholic.

While this model can be helpful, in one important way it fails to encompass and explain the whole of the causation of alcoholism. Although it works clinically, it is useful only for explaining why alcoholism develops in a particular individual. It does not account for the widespread existence of alcoholism or for its occurrence at differing rates in different population, age and sex groups. People, after all, have their various personalities, and most of us are beset by difficult life problems at some time or other. The weakness of the model is that if we regard drinking merely as the device that some people use, perhaps almost fortuitously, to cope with their problems, we neglect the fundamental role of alcohol in causing alcoholism.

And so we turn to the last of the four theories, whose central point is that there can be no alcoholism without alcohol. Moreover, the more alcohol there is about, the greater will be the number of alcoholics. This is the new feature for which conclusive evidence has come to light only relatively recently. Of course it must seem obvious. The more people drink, the more alcoholics there will be. The implications are significant, since the corollary is that the more you and I drink, the more that each of us drinks socially, the more alcoholics shall thereby be created. If the facts are correct then the drinking habits of each one of us influence

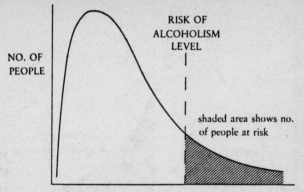

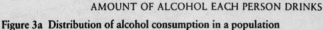

Figure 3a Distribution of alcohol consumption in a population

the extent of alcoholism in our community. Put starkly like that it becomes much less obvious that there is a relationship between the total amount of alcohol consumed by any population and the number of alcoholics there will be. We now have abundant proof. In every country where the matter has been studied, the total amount of alcohol consumed bears a close relationship to the number of alcoholics. Whatever index of alcoholic harm we care to take, physical, psychological or social, whether it be deaths from liver disease, admissions to medical wards with physical illnesses or to psychiatric wards with mental illnesses due to alcoholism, convictions for drunken driving, or arrests for drunkenness offences, the rates of these rise when the total sales of alcoholic beverages rise. We can make the comparison between countries with high and low consumption rates or in one country over time as consumption rates vary; it always holds. Alcohol in the clinical model may be merely a device; when an epidemiologist considers a large population, he observes that it is alcohol which causes alcoholism.

The distribution of drinking within a population assumes the form shown in Figure 3a.

Those individuals who come on the right-hand side of the graph, that is, those who are drinking a great deal, say more than 15 gms of absolute alcohol a day, are highly at risk of developing

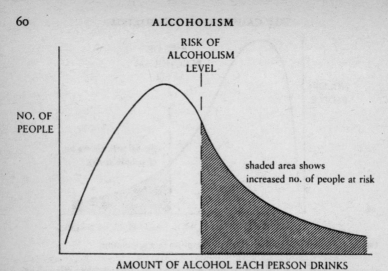

Figure 3b **Distribution of alcohol consumption in the same population after increased overall consumption**

alcoholism. If the whole population drinks more the graph changes shape, as in Figure 3b, and the number of people at risk of developing alcoholism is increased.

The connection between price going down (relative to total amount of earnings) and consumption rising is shown in Figure 4, which also shows that when consumption rises so do the indices of alcoholism.

We have unfortunately to take the matter one stage further; unfortunately because it presents all of us with an unavoidable moral dilemma. Various factors determine how much alcohol a given society will consume. There can be cultural, ethnic or religious proscriptions upon both drinking and excessive drinking, there can be laws regulating the hours of sale, the number of outlets for sale per head of population, the age of permitted drinking and the amount that we can bring into the country duty free. All these have an effect, especially the licensing laws. Overwhelmingly, however, the factor that chiefly influences consumption is price. When drink becomes cheaper, more is sold, and drunk; raise the price and consumption falls. The data show how close is the relationship. So, should we urge an increase in price, and

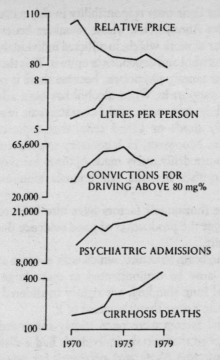

Figure 4 Alcohol: Price, consumption and related harms in the UK

possibly also a decrease in availability, in order to reduce the number of alcoholics? We shall return to this when considering the prevention of alcoholism. Meanwhile it will be necessary, later in this chapter, to try to integrate this epidemiological model with the clinical model described earlier.

Physical Causes

Before that, we need to consider some of the theories that have been put forward to explain why this person does and that person does not become an alcoholic. It has been postulated that there are physical differences between individuals to account for this. Such a view is very comforting to alcoholics, who need not, therefore, consider their own responsibility in the matter. It is taken by Alcoholics Anonymous, whose members believe there is an allergic factor at work which, in afflicted individuals, causes both craving for alcohol and dependence upon it. This theory has never found favour among physicians, because there is no convincing evidence to support it. When alcohol has been administered to alcoholics they show none of the characteristic reactions, in the tissues, body fluids or blood cells, that indicate an allergic phenomenon. Moreover, in laboratory experiments where the conditions were deliberately made optimal for showing allergic responses, neither humans nor animals manifested such responses.

Endocrine (hormonal) factors have also been suggested but, again, without the production of good evidence that they play a causative part.

Changes in brain structure, which with modern scanning techniques can now be demonstrated in quite large numbers of alcoholics of long standing, are rightly considered to be due to the alcoholism rather than the cause of it.

Nutritional factors were once widely canvassed. One set of theories implied that certain individuals had a dietary lack of a specific factor (the N_1 factor) necessary for metabolism. Rats whose diets lacked this factor were found, it was claimed, to take more alcohol than other rats. Later experimental work has cast very considerable doubt on what may be concluded from such observations.

Another theory is that alcoholics inherit an enzyme abnormality which, because it impairs metabolism of certain substances, increases the need for them and thus sets up a metabolic pattern predisposed to alcoholism. Although some of the research behind this theory has been carried out on alcoholics, there is no warrant for the belief that any metabolic disorder is inherited or indeed that it preceded the alcoholism. This last objection applies to many theories which postulate physical factors operating *before* excessive drinking develops. Craving for alcohol, or dependence on it, has not been shown to occur before drinking has taken place, yet many of the theories would require this if they were to be substantiated.

Theories where the pathological or biochemical or endocrinological changes are presumed to be subsequent to heavy drinking but then act to make it get out of control are more plausible. The setting-in of brain damage is very likely to be such a factor. Equally, social disabilities that result from excessive drinking can act to increase the drinking, and it is obvious that when dependence develops it must lead, in its turn, to increased drinking. We shall use such arguments shortly to produce a rounded theory of causation.

The method of inheritance of alcoholism is very complex. There is no doubt at all that alcoholism can run in families. Sons of alcoholics have a much higher incidence of alcoholism than other men of the same age. But that does not mean that alcoholism is inherited in a biological way. After all, sons of rich men tend to be much richer than sons of other men. There is a difference between familial inheritance and inheritance through the genes. Whether a tendency to alcohol is inherited genetically, rather than by example or by another form of cultural transmission, is not known for sure. Some studies have shown that children of alcoholic parents, adopted virtually at birth by non-alcoholic parents, have a higher incidence of becoming alcoholic than children of non-alcoholic parents, similarly adopted. This certainly suggests biological transmission. On the other hand, studies of the incidence of alcoholism in identical, compared with non-identical, twins of alcoholics have not yielded clear-cut answers, nor have studies of identical twins reared apart. If there is genetical inheritance of alcoholism it certainly does not follow any simple inheritance rules, so it must be polygenic rather than following a straightforward pattern of dominant or recessive inheritance of a single gene. We know little of the way in which personality is genetically determined, though enough to be certain that cultural and environmental factors by themselves are not the sole determinants. Possibly, therefore, transmission of a tendency to alcoholism could be linked to the inheritance of personality, itself a complex matter.

Some writers have suggested that any genetic transmission of alcoholism that there may be occurs through the known genetic inheritance of depressive illness which can produce alcoholism in some people. According to this view, the inherited factor of depression may be sufficient to account for the inheritance of alcoholism.

However, in our own view, while there may possibly be some genetic transmission of alcoholism, the non-genetic, familial, aspect of heavy drinking in the parental home having its effect on the child, by way of example, is a much more potent factor. Familial but not genetically inherited factors can work in a paradoxical way. If parents have strong views disapproving of drinking, then a rebellious adolescent or young adult may turn to excessive drinking as a way of revolt.

The present state of knowledge permits no authoritative statement concerning the mode of inheritance of alcoholism (though of course that does not prevent dogmatic assertions being made). Nevertheless, we know that children of alcoholics are at increased risk of becoming alcoholics themselves, just as we know that daughters of alcoholics are more likely to marry alcoholics, and for that there can be no genetic explanation.

Social Causes

Two of the social and cultural causes of alcoholism have already been mentioned. The first is opportunity: the availability of alcohol. This is linked chiefly with price but also with ease of access, that is, the number of places where it can be bought. The number of these outlets per head of population is rising fast. Access is also made easier if the hours of permitted sale are increased. Most countries of the world do not have laws or regulations limiting the hours when drink may be sold. In Great Britain, however, the number of hours is limited. An increase in permitted hours was made recently in Scotland; England and Wales followed suit in August 1988. There is also the question of the age at which youths can enter bars, etc., to purchase drinks. Supply is the parent of opportunity. It is this aspect that accounts for the relatively high extent of alcoholism among those who work in the drink or entertainments trades, and among the better off.

The second factor is example, where not only parental drinking is influential, but also drinking by others on whom young people are liable to model themselves: their peers, and perhaps more important, sportsmen and women, pop stars, television and screen personalities and the characters they portray.

A third factor is incitement. The pressure of advertising, on television, on hoardings and in the printed media is relentless, and we return to this in Chapter 13.

Cultural attitudes towards alcoholism and drinking are also potent factors. Our society as a whole does not look askance at drunkenness, does not regard driving while over the legal limit as a particularly heinous matter ('haven't we all done it?'). Our society tends to view drinking as a manly business and looks with a hint of prejudice at men who do not drink. Female drinking is on the increase. This may merely reflect greater female affluence but may it not also contain an element of emulation? Within Britain, the Scots drink more than the English, Catholics more than members of other Christian denominations, Asians and Jews relatively little. To link the epidemiological picture with the clinical model explaining the forces acting on particular individuals, we need to consider how it may be that someone who comes (it might be by chance, though not necessarily so) to be on the right-hand side of the distribution curve of drinking in the population goes on to become an alcoholic.

For all other medical conditions, the condition itself has a recognizable set of causes and a set of recognizable consequences. For alcoholism the causes and the consequences are one and the same. Those features that arise as a result of heavy drinking are the very features that give rise to such drinking. Thus a vicious circle is set up, or rather, as we shall see, four vicious circles, seemingly separate but in fact interlocking.

The simplest of these is the vicious circle of dependence. If excessive drinkers, as a result of the drinking, become dependent on alcohol, then they will have to go on drinking more and more, and, in turn, the extent of the excessive drinking increases.

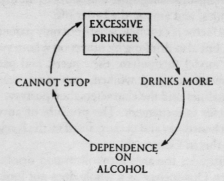

Figure 5a Vicious circle of dependence

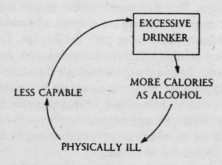

Figure 5b Vicious circle of bodily damage

The next vicious circle is of bodily damage. The excessive drinker starts to take a very high proportion of daily calorie intake as alcohol. This is likely to lead to the development of some sort of bodily damage. A consequence is that the alcohol dependant becomes less able, more helpless, and continues to drink even more out of a sense of personal weakness.

The third of these vicious circles concerns the social predica-

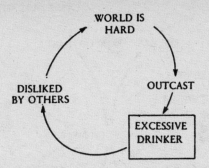

Figure 5c Vicious circle of social predicament

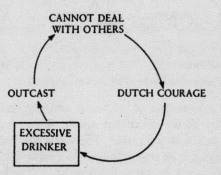

Figure 5d Psychological vicious circle

ments that alcoholics may find themselves in. Because of the excessive drinking, people do not like them. They find the world hard and, indeed, it begins to cast them out, to dismiss them from work, to exclude them from invitations and so on. To compensate for this they drink even more.

The final circle is a psychological one. Excessive drinkers feel themselves to be outcasts. They cannot successfully deal with others. So they drink to bolster their attempts to remain psychologically adept, what we sometimes call Dutch courage, and so the drinking mounts.

Using these models we begin to understand why those who start to drink more than their fellows may come to escalate their

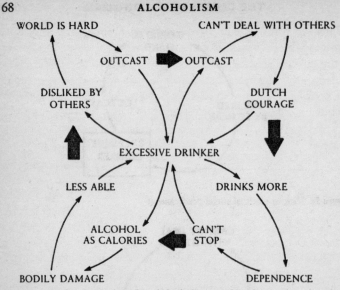

WORLD IS HARD   CAN'T DEAL WITH OTHERS

OUTCAST   OUTCAST

DISLIKED BY   DUTCH
OTHERS   COURAGE

EXCESSIVE DRINKER

LESS ABLE   DRINKS MORE

ALCOHOL   CAN'T
AS CALORIES   STOP

BODILY DAMAGE   DEPENDENCE

Figure 6 The four vicious circles of alcoholism combined

drinking. But in respect of the social and psychological vicious circles it may be the other way round. This takes us back to the clinical model stated earlier. The social predicaments, or the inability, arising from psychological deficits, to deal with people, might have caused the excessive drinking in the first place, but equally, the drinking to excess could have led to the difficulties, and so on. The vicious circles, therefore, embrace both the epidemiological and clinical models. Nor is this all. Each of these vicious circles will itself increase drinking, but if we put them all together we can see how one easily leads to another.

Once drinkers cannot stop (the dependency circle), they inevitably take a higher and higher proportion of their daily calorie intake as alcohol so they are likely to get into the bodily damage circle; once they become less able, people will like them less (the social predicaments circle); once they are cast out they are even more likely to regard themselves as outcasts and so be within the psychological circle. All this happens because those things which are the consequences of excessive drinking act as the cause of even more drinking.

When we come later to consider treatment we shall see how the two models of alcoholism each show the way to understanding the principles of treatment: dealing with the person, the problems and the device of alcohol that they have chosen to help them cope with the problems, thus breaking the vicious circles in which the alcoholic has become trapped.

Chapter 7

Varieties of Drinking Pattern

The drinking patterns of alcoholics can take widely varying forms. In this chapter we shall be discussing what types of drinking pattern we can recognize and the usefulness of distinguishing between them.

Some writers on alcoholism, particularly influenced by Alcoholics Anonymous, have tended to concentrate exclusively upon one pattern of drinking (which we shall be describing under the heading of the compulsive alcoholic) and to ignore the many other distinct forms that are to be found. So many members of Alcoholics Anonymous drink in this pattern that to them it is the paradigm of alcoholism. As Jellinek[17] put it, 'Alcoholics Anonymous have naturally created the picture of alcoholism in their own image.' This narrow approach does a serious disservice. There are many people who have to be classified as alcoholics and need treatment on that basis, but whose drinking is not of the compulsive variety. Otherwise errors will be made both in the provision and planning of treatment and in turning away people who are motivated for treatment and would be eminently responsive.

A close examination of the drinking pattern makes possible much more than the mere recognition that a person is an alcoholic. Getting a careful account of the mode of drinking is essential for correct assessment of the individual's problem, and on this depends the treatment regime which will be advised.

The Unsuspecting Alcoholic

Many people drink themselves into alcoholism without perceiving that they are addicted. They may not have any conspicuous abnormality of personality. Sometimes, and this is far from being uncommon, people have a physical illness or injury the nature or circumstances of which prompt (or should prompt) the doctor to question them about drinking. They may have broken a leg and appeared intoxicated at hospital; they may have a gastric ulcer or another condition of which alcohol is known frequently to be the cause; one or more of the easily recognized complications of alcoholism may be evident, such as cirrhosis of the liver or peripheral neuritis. Questioning, if it be pursued, might reveal three things: that these people regularly consume a great deal of alcohol, that they never considered themselves as alcoholics and that they had not before had any trouble from drinking. The physician or surgeon who views the task primarily as that of treating the physical disorder should go on to diagnose the underlying alcoholism, but may be inclined to leave the interrogation there; the patient is then thought of as someone who is the victim of alcohol without being affected by alcoholism. Alternatively, the patient may be recognized as an alcoholic but the management of this aspect of the condition is not pursued. The notion of being an alcoholic or being dependent on alcohol would be vigorously dismissed if it were put to the patient. But it is not. The physician's disinclination to explore the diagnosis is strengthened if the patient does not show any craving for alcohol while being treated. Only if the patient asks for alcohol or shows withdrawal symptoms will the true nature of the dependence become apparent.

We have discussed in the previous chapters the factors that contribute to the development of alcoholism. It rarely develops purely by mischance: predisposing factors in the individual are the rule. Appropriate interviewing techniques will generally elicit first from such patients that if they do not have a drink their equanimity and poise is sufficiently disturbed to prevent them carrying on smoothly with life. It is likely also to reveal the very important matter that there have been occasions when they have become fearful of the hold alcohol has gained on them, and have tried to give it up. In spite of their protestations that on discharge they will effortlessly stop drinking, they seldom do so. Most of these people have insidiously become dependent on alcohol, but because they have acquired a high tolerance they have rarely appeared blatantly intoxicated. Consequently they may not come to medical notice until nutritional disorders develop. These may be hastened by dietary restrictions due to economic stringency. It is a great disservice to allow such people to leave hospital unacquainted with the reality of their situation. A few of them may manage to give up drinking by their own efforts, but for the great majority special attention is essential if they are not to continue to deteriorate. Alcoholics cannot go for long without drinking. Once away from the sheltered environment that hospital provides they revert to abnormal drinking.

An accountant aged forty was admitted to hospital with a gastric ulcer. At that time he was drinking two bottles of whisky a day. This was noted as a cause for his ulcer, and he was advised to cut down. When he was told why, he cheerfully assented. However, when he left hospital he found himself unable to do so. Eight months later he had an attack of delirium tremens. Even after this he could not accept that he was an alcoholic. It was only after a subsequent suicide attempt that he consented to enter hospital for the treatment of alcoholism. Evidence of a lifelong personality abnormality was then revealed. As a child, if he was called on to perform at school or at parties he would weep. As a young man he could speak in public only if he drank beforehand. Towards his mother, and subsequently towards his wife, he was both excessively aggressive and abnormally dependent. In the therapeutic situation he at first attempted to evade exploration of his behaviour by adopting a manner of jaunty superficiality. When this was penetrated he became seriously involved in his own treatment.

The Regular but Restrained Alcoholic

We use this term to describe alcoholics who must drink every day. Their daily consumption may be considerable, but they are not forced to finish all their supplies or to exhaust their money. To this extent, therefore, they are able to regulate their excessive drinking, and under the pressure of extraordinary social demands they may be able to take less than their normal wont. Nevertheless, such people are not likely to go for as long as a day without a drink and, as the condition progresses, they will always take a drink first thing in the morning. They cannot tolerate being sober but rarely need to drink to the point of drunkenness. It is characteristic of this type of drinker that they can control the amount they take in at any one time. This variety of alcoholism has classically been called 'inability to abstain'.

If the person stops drinking, voluntarily or because obliged to, craving will appear, and it is almost certain that there will be withdrawal symptoms. There is not only psychological dependence, therefore, but physical dependence as well, the result of continued excessive drinking. The patient has acquired tissue tolerance.

People who drink regularly in a bar with the same group of friends are a well-recognized variant. They compensate in this way for deficiencies in their other social relationships. Everywhere else they feel inferior; only here, surrounded by trusted and uncritical companions, increasingly so as the evening proceeds, are they able to feel at ease, inspired by the fellow-feeling which the group engenders. Drink follows drink, round after round; each drinker orders in turn, not only for the satisfaction of their own drink but also for the pleasure they get from treating the friends they hold in such regard. Here at least they are somebody's peer.

Some who drink excessively in a group in a bar are in fact isolated, friendless people. Passive, good-natured, unambitious, they have never learned from mature relationships; and in the undemanding, casual camaraderie of the bar they are never taxed intellectually or emotionally. They are in their element.

These drinkers regularly consume a considerable quantity of alcohol in the course of an evening, yet because they do not hurry over it, and because they have had many years to acquire tolerance, they rarely show gross intoxication.

Gregarious drinkers are there for all to see. Equally so are some solitary drinkers. It is common in public houses to find people sitting by themselves at a table or at a corner of the bar steadily drinking hour after hour and clearly disinclined to engage in or be engaged in any social intercourse. Morose, unheeding of their surroundings, they are conducting the business of drinking without the interference of conversation. They choose to drink in the pub rather than at home because they escape the family's antagonism and because the pub is geared to dispense their supplies with the minimum of inconvenience.

Other solitary drinkers drink at home. If they are women they will generally do this in secret. Both men and women secret drinkers like to foster an image of sobriety, and dissemble desperately when suspected. Home drinkers generally drink every day. They cannot abstain longer, but the quantity stays under control: they do not get drunk. Women who are at home while their husbands are at work often make a pathetic attempt each evening to hide the evidence of their drinking. Their plight is extreme. Regrettably, when alcoholics, particularly women, drink secretly, it is difficult for anyone to penetrate the secrecy, gain their confidence and help them to get expert help. The forty-year-old woman living down the road and drinking three bottles of sherry a day that Edwards[18] described, is, alas, on her own with her drinking. Edwards asks what can be done to initiate humane, technically competent and integrated help . . . before the liver is damaged, children are in care or suicide is considered? But if no one knows about their drinking, no one can help.

The Compulsive Alcoholic

A different variety of alcoholism is that occurring in people who, once they have started to drink, cannot stop but must go on until all their money is spent or their supplies are finished or until accident or unconsciousness supervene. Such drinkers can have abstinent periods, but as soon as they begin to drink again they cannot limit the quantity. This pattern has been aptly named 'loss of control'. In mild cases the amount of drink taken may gradually increase for several days after a period of abstinence. Eventually, however, the point of drunkenness is reached.

Another variant, which stops short of the full picture, occurs when some self-restraint can operate although drunkenness has been reached; the alcoholic retains sufficient foresight and manages to desist in spite of there being drink still available. A married schoolteacher of forty-five worked for five days each week without drinking. Every Friday as soon as school ended she would start drinking gin to such an extent that by nightfall she was very intoxicated, very outgoing and talking excessively. She misbehaved socially and abused her husband, accusing him of paying her too little attention. Next morning she would be unaware of the disturbance she had caused in her own and her friends' homes. She continued to drink during Saturday and became drunk and forgetful once more; on Sunday morning she would wake feeling remorseful and apprehensive, and although she began to drink straight away she was able to go to school and do her work in the ensuing week. She was more fortunate than most of those who suffer from loss of control. They are powerless to prevent their spells from going on to prolonged drunkenness. Invariably they suffer from withdrawal symptoms, for they have become physiologically dependent on alcohol, and it is very common for them not to be able to remember the later events of the spell of drinking even though they did not lose consciousness.

Compulsive alcoholics are the mainstay of Alcoholics Anonymous. It is easy to see how they have developed the idea that alcohol is a specific poison for them, on the basis of a prior physical sensitivity. The view is incorrect; but, since the alcoholic later becomes physiologically dependent, the idea that alcohol is a poison may help sustain the struggle for abstinence.

Between bouts of drinking, compulsive alcoholics may remain abstinent for periods of some days. A stranger meeting them at such a time would not discern that they were dependent upon alcohol. Although this type of alcoholic finds temporary sobriety bearable, as soon as they have one drink a train of events is set in motion. They are compelled to continue drinking until their physical reactions, some serious disease or injury, or mounting terror of the consequences if they continue, forces them to stop. The alcoholic caught up in this furious progress can no longer freely choose between leaving off or continuing to drink.

Alcoholics who drink in this pattern get into serious social difficulties. Their drunken behaviour repels. They alienate and antagonize those who come into contact with them, even when these people are anxious to be helpful.

The Neurotic Alcoholic

The alcoholics described so far in this chapter do not suffer from additional clear-cut psychological illnesses. But alcoholism can be the most evident disturbance in a patient whose principal disorder is, in fact, neurosis. The alcoholism is not primary, and the form of the drinking is not distinctive. Very varied patterns are adopted. Alcoholics with neurosis drink to reduce their subjective distress, to diminish their emotional conflicts. Their drinking represents an attempt to cure the symptoms of the underlying condition. However, as the level of drinking usually exceeds what is acceptable socially, it worsens their inter-personal situation. They then use alcohol to try to counteract the symptoms which stem from disturbed inter-personal relationships, but unfortunately their friends and relatives have to put up with the added embarrassments of the drinking superimposed on the pre-existing psychological difficulties. So the drinking is self-defeating. Yet they may persist in it for many years, knowing no alternative. Physical dependence develops in time, with resultant addiction. However, if proper attention is paid to the underlying psychological disorder, the alcoholism may be relinquished by the patient. The treatment in such a case must aim to deal with the psychological disorder, but effective therapeutic impact on the patient, by either individual psychotherapy or group therapy, to deal with the neurosis is not possible until the drinking has been interrupted.

Symptomatic Alcoholism

Sometimes alcoholism occurs in a patient already suffering from a severe psychiatric disorder. This must then take first place in management. Alcoholism can be the symptom which brings to notice people suffering from depression or schizophrenia, from psychiatric illness due to brain disease or from mental subnormality.

The physician who treats numbers of alcoholics will always be on the look-out to detect the patient whose drinking should properly be regarded only as a symptom of severe underlying psychiatric illness, the diagnosis of which calls for careful history-taking and psychiatric examination.

A sixty-year-old unmarried businesswoman had retired. For forty years she had cared for her mother whom she described as a very determined person, the decision-maker in the family despite her constant laziness. In addition to being selfish, the mother distressed the family by always wanting to be at whist-drives, parties or the theatre. She had been widowed early, and in her old age deteriorated mentally; she had bowel trouble and soiled in the house. Six months previously her daughter, the patient, became depressed, felt unable to relax and slept poorly; she did not know what to do about her mother and resentfully thought that the old lady just did not care about controlling her bowel movements. She began to drink heavily, soon taking half a bottle of brandy every day and a good deal of sherry. The drink did not relieve her depression but gave her the necessary energy to attack the added washing as well as the household chores. A month before she was first seen for her alcoholism the family doctor arranged for her mother to enter a home. The patient became still more depressed. She felt like a lost soul, increasingly sad and sleepless. She realized that she could not stop drinking. 'I think I'm an alcoholic. I don't think I'll be able to control my drinking even if I get better from this depression. Everybody says I shouldn't feel guilty about putting my mother away but I should have been able to cope until she was finished. It's duty rather than love.' She had used alcohol to boost herself up, to help her get some sleep, to reduce her restlessness and to ease the distress of 'worrying too much about things I needn't worry about'.

This patient's condition was a depressive illness originally centred on her resentment towards her mother; her sense of failure and self-blame when her mother had to be sent away were other symptoms of the illness. The alcoholism was secondary to the psychiatric disorder, and drug treatment for her depression with psychotherapeutic measures was successful. She recovered quickly and proceeded to arrange a long cruise for herself. Drinking was no longer a problem to her.

Alcoholism may also be seen occasionally as an early manifestation of the psychoses caused by organic diseases of the brain or as part of the general picture of senile mental deterioration. In this group with structural brain lesions, the drinking tends to be both purposeless and poorly organized.

Bout Drinkers

We have left to the last an unusual drinking pattern which is not classifiable into any of the previous groups.

There are people who for three to six months, and sometimes longer, drink only socially, if at all. They then suddenly start to drink excessively, for days on end, drinking all the time, neglecting all their responsibilities at work or to their families. Sometimes they do serious damage to themselves or to others during the bouts. Days or weeks later they just as suddenly stop.

A forty-five-year-old male schoolteacher drank excessively in bouts of two to three days, with approximately four months between each bout. The longest gap was fourteen months.

Ordinarily I never have more than a sherry. Once I start drinking more, just civilized social drinking, it brings the possibility of a bout nearer reality. I know when one is imminent. I think to myself, 'I'm going to get drunk tonight and, God, how I dread it.' When I start up, there seems to be a determined attitude to get really stinko, plastered. I'm determined then to stay drunk for forty-eight hours to three days, until I get into a thoroughly toxic state. All that will keep me quiet is more alcohol. Only drugs can get me out of the cycle, which I badly want to come to an end. I've never lost a job, but I've had to be hospitalized a number of times. It's almost as if a bout is unconsciously planned. It happens when I feel: 'Now I can let go, escape from things'. First there's the build-up, then the letting go. I have a spurt of 'you only live once, to hell with it'. It's a wild, exuberant, thoughtless, throw-it-down. I weep for my wife in many respects. I honestly don't know what the solution is. I don't know what to do about myself now.

For many months a bout drinker may be untroubled by any urge to drink and, in fact, may have been able to drink socially; but once the bout starts it progresses relentlessly. A shopkeeper was seen after he had suffered from periodic drinking bouts for thirty years. He came for treatment because he felt that he could no longer bear the physical consequences of a drinking bout:

> I get jittery, especially when I am trying to stop. What annoys me is that I can last for as long as ten months, but then it all starts up again. First I have an urge to start for two or three days, set off by fortuitous happenings, a drink advertisement which catches my eye or a brewery wagon passing. Then I succumb. I feel guilty about it soon after I have started, because I am a disgrace to my family. My daughter ignores me lately and she comes home late from school because she is sick of the sight of me; she wants to stay out of the house as much as possible, rather than face the sight of me.

The great interest of bout drinking stems from this alternation of brief but grossly pathological drinking with long phases of normality. Periodic drinkers of this sort usually deny that any particular psychological stress is required to trigger off the drinking phases, nor can upsetting events be incriminated. This unusual form of drinking used to be called dipsomania or periodic alcoholism.

We have seen that the various patterns of abnormal drinking can be associated with disorders of personality (most cases come in this category), with underlying neurotic illness or with psychoses or underlying brain disease. Each of these characteristically sets up its own form of pathological use of alcohol and each requires a separate method of management. The global term of alcoholism is used to cover them all. But their clinical examination must include a careful process of differentiation to determine the category in which a particular person's drinking belongs.

Chapter 8

Stages in Being an Alcoholic

Every alcoholic's history is unique. Personal experiences, psychological disturbances, social shifts and upheavals, physical illnesses and changes in drinking habits all contribute to a sequence of events particular to each individual. But the student of alcoholism, who meets similar phenomena over and over again in different patients, discerns customary progressions. The alcoholic's total career spans successive periods of illness, each with its own phases which can be identified by their characteristic symptoms as they proceed. Some events generally take place early; others feature in the later stages of the condition. The order in which we shall describe them is derived from considering large numbers of alcoholics; no particular patient will be found who follows it exactly. Events which typically occur early in the course may be found late in the histories of some alcoholics or may never be seen at all. Some patients pass with dramatic rapidity from the early stages of alcoholism to the severest levels with scarcely any intermediate phase. There are individual variations of considerable magnitude. The ensuing outline of a step-like series of phases represents only a composite picture; nevertheless it is faithful to the generality of alcoholics. The alcoholic begins with excessive drinking, moves into the stage of dependence, and progresses to reach the stage of chronic alcoholism with physical and mental breakdown. Two transitions have special significance. The first of these, which marks the onset of alcoholism, occurs when a person is no longer just an excessive drinker but has become harmed. The second, when the alcoholic passes into chronic alcoholism, is marked by the development of severe and persistent bodily changes.

Phases in Alcoholism

Stage of Excessive Drinking

More time spent in social drinking

Drinks more nights of the week

Sneaks drinks

Takes stronger drinks than companions

Adopts strategies to get more drinks

Preoccupied with drinking

Drinks to get relief from tension

Increased tolerance

Guilt over drinking

Social failures excused with fabricated explanations

Needs drinks to perform adequately at work or socially

Feels drink has become a necessity

Increased guilt feelings

Stage of Alcohol Dependence

Onset of alcohol amnesias (memory losses)

Greater frequency of amnesias

Loss of control – compulsive drinking

Reduction in interests

Drop in work efficiency

Absenteeism

Drunk in the daytime

Reproof from employer or relatives

Low self-esteem

Remorse

Compensatory bragging and generosity

Financial extravagance

Deceives family, debts made

Increasing social isolation

Aggressive outbursts

Spouse takes over more responsibilities

Deterioration in family relations

Paranoid misinterpretations

Self-pity

Justifies drinking with self-deceptions

Reduction of sexual drive

Morbid jealousy

Drunk at week-ends

Loss of job

Break-up of family

Morning tremulousness

Morning drinking

Conceals supplies of liquor

Repeated attempts to stop drinking

Suicidal impulses and attempts

Neglect of meals

Stage of Chronic Alcoholism

Physical and mental symptoms dominate

Loss of appetite, poor food intake

Continuous drinking

Tolerance diminishes

Prolonged confused thinking

Use of cheap wines and methylated spirits

Delirium tremens

Goes to A A or seeks medical treatment

Serious physical diseases

Excessive Drinking

In the early stages of abnormal drinking, although excessive drinkers take more alcohol than normal social drinkers, they drink in the same pattern. There are nevertheless warning signs that excessive drinking has developed. Not only is the person drinking more than other people; he or she, and this is very important, is drinking more than formerly. *More time is spent drinking*, more nights of the week and more hours each night. It may not be long before the person finds that sufficient drink cannot be obtained by drinking in a socially accepted manner, and *sneaking drinks* begins. This involves drinking round for round with friends but also obtaining additional drinks between the rounds.

Stratagems are also adopted to get still more drink while disguising this from others. Companions may be left for a moment on some pretext while a quick drink is consumed at a different bar. Or the alcoholic may go from bar to bar in succession so that the acquaintance met in any one will not realize the amount being imbibed. At home, the pale liquid in his or her own glass may be whisky and not the sherry poured for everybody else. Visits to the kitchen are not always to get ice. In other people's houses alcoholics do not take long to discover where the strong drink can be found and will not be backward in pouring their own. A number of preparatory drinks will have been taken before arriving at one's host's, and if it is calculated that there will not be enough drink there, one can bring along some of one's own.

All these devices manifest an *avidity for alcohol* and a determination to get the quantity which the alcoholic now requires. This is done without shame, because one is not yet aware what these actions portend. Alcoholics do not see themselves as marked out from their fellows even though the necessity is there to conceal drinking from friends in case they are beginning to notice.

Drinking at this stage affords positive relief. The alcoholic has discovered that the taking of alcohol lessens tension. 'I was shy at dances and had a drink to relax me and make me more sociable. It gave me the courage to dance. I could not have done it without drink.' He felt better for drinking. Having *discovered that alcohol brings relief*, the excessive drinker now uses it for this end nearly every day and becomes a regular drinker.

This increase in drinking results in an *increased tolerance* for alcohol, so that a given amount of drink has less effect. Although having to drink more to obtain the relief sought for, alcoholics may be quite cheered by this. They can take the amount needed and yet stay fairly sober. They may even congratulate themselves upon their ability to hold their liquor. What is taking place, however, is a physiological change, an alteration in the body's reaction to alcohol. Round about this time, the first two or three *drinks may be consumed with great rapidity* in order to get the effect as quickly as possible. The person begins to feel different from other people, separate from friends whose unspoken objection is sensed. Certain friends will deliberately be avoided, contact being broken off with those whose criticisms have been or would be most distressing. Paradoxically, this is part of an uphill and futile attempt to preserve oneself socially by remaining only in the company of those who are unconcerned because they are less closely associated personally. Excuses are invented for missed opportunities and unfulfilled promises. Alcoholics dislike themselves for being deceitful. They know now that they are covering up. They are beginning to be *assailed by guilt* about what they are having to do in order to get the drink they need.

The stage has been reached where it is felt that, to function properly, there is an imperative need for the effects of alcohol. A drink has to be taken to prepare oneself for routine activities.

Alcohol Dependence

Drinking is now a necessity. Drink is now being taken not so much for pleasure as to experience its effects. The alcoholic, for such the person now indubitably is, frequently *drinks to the point of drunkenness*. Inevitably this has its physical consequences. *Losses of memory occur*. On recovery from a drinking session there is no memory for its later stages. In such a situation, alcoholics cannot say how they got home, nor remember whether they disgraced themselves. In reality the behaviour has generally been unexceptionable. The first intimation to friends may be an anxious and devious probing next day to discover how they had acted. Lack of awareness during the drinking is not responsible for the blank: the appropriateness of the behaviour at the time proves this. There is no possibility of later recall of what transpired because no record of the events was stored in the memory. It is no use cudgelling one's brains to remember: there is no imprint there to be recalled.

Alcoholics are sometimes too shocked at the first occurrence of such an amnesia to admit to themselves that a whole sequence of experience has not been remembered. One described how disconcerted he was at receiving a letter from a business associate, dealing with a telephone conversation this man had had with the patient: 'I can remember no such conversation. I'm a bit worried that I may have forgotten. But I doubt that. Perhaps it was a mythical telephone conversation that he was referring to.'

Such memory blanks may occur in excessive drinkers even at times when they have not been drinking particularly heavily. Some patients can tell you accurately when they first started. 'By then I would have a couple of drinks during the day and really hit it at night. I often awoke in the morning unable to remember what had happened during parts of the previous day.' Almost all can remember their first episode even if they cannot date it. Amnesic spells are particularly alarming if the alcoholic fears that someone might have been done serious harm but cannot remember if this is the case. This happened to a young machine operator. His wife said that one night he came in late in a very distressed state and with blood on his hands, shirt and underclothes. He was unable to remember where he had been and what he had been doing. Later he made inquiries and discovered that a girl at work had left the factory with him and they had had sexual intercourse. It might have taken place, he thought, in a forest or park, but his memory went no further.

The term 'blackout' is often used to describe this amnesia, particularly by alcoholics themselves, but it is misleading because there has been no unconsciousness. The abnormality is a failure to register events in the memory. Physical changes in brain activity are responsible for this extraordinary phenomenon, which nearly all alcoholics have experienced. Upon them the effect is shattering: they can no longer hide from themselves that they are being harmed by drink. It is at the blackout stage that many alcoholics first seek help. To the physician they are a clear sign that, without treatment, reversion to moderate, controlled drinking is unlikely, and the patient is set on an inexorable downhill course. When the *frequency of amnesias increases*, so that memory blanks become quite regular and they occur not as isolated and shocking events but as repeated aspects of drinking life, another milestone has been reached.

Once the person dependent on alcohol begins to lose the power either to decide in advance how much to drink or to stick to that decision, *the capacity to regulate drinking has become lost*. Such alcoholics repeatedly find themselves in the position of taking more than they meant to; this phenomenon is designated by the phrase 'loss of control'. The alcoholic has become a compulsive drinker. One drink leads inevitably to a succession of others despite the extreme inappropriateness of such behaviour. At its worst, this loss in control means that each time the alcoholic starts to drink, he or she will continue until helpless.

Drinking now takes up the greater part of the alcoholic's time, thoughts and energy, and thus *interests become narrower*. An evening at the cinema is an evening's drinking lost. An employer may notice a *loss of working efficiency*: errors creep in, sales go down; unpunctuality and short periods of *absenteeism* occur. (In firms which seek to identify and treat alcoholics, works managers are taught to recognize Monday-morning absenteeism as a likely sign of alcoholism.) Even when at work, the alcoholic may be inattentive, and forgetfulness may have serious consequences. Inevitably there will come a day when he or she is clearly the worse for drink while at work. Being *drunk in the daytime* has begun. 'I wasn't sober for the last five months of my army service,' was how an ex-soldier described the occurrence of such daytime drunkenness.

All those with whom alcoholics have contact, relatives, friends, work-mates and employers, are remonstrating or reprimanding. They warn that unless there is a mending of ways they will take action. These *increasing social pressures* make the alcoholic's position more insecure and exacerbate the drinking.

Self-esteem at this stage is very low. The alcoholics regard themselves as worthless and despicable. They may be tempted to misdemeanours by the overriding need for drink:

> At first I'd go to the cash-box only to take change, to put a five-pound note in and take five single pounds out. Then I began taking money out to spend on drink, with the idea of replacing it on pay-day. Lately, replacing the money was my last consideration.

They are *beset with remorse* at the way they have let themselves and everyone else down. To compensate, they may resort to *dwelling on past achievements*, sometimes exaggerating them in a grandiose way to impress those who are still prepared to tolerate their company. They may tell gross lies to put themselves in a better light.

> When I first met my wife I told her my right hand was weak because of a combat injury. Really it was due to polio. I also told her I was five years older than my true age. After telling these lies I was obsessed with the idea that my wife might discover about the polio and leave me or that her father might ask me a question about the army and make my lies apparent.

To lend credibility to such tales of worthiness and success they may *spend large amounts of money* in treating others with undue ostentation. It is not uncommon for a person to walk into a pub with a full week's wages and leave penniless later in the evening.

An alcoholic may attempt to recover losses by ill-judged speculations and may frequently resort to gambling in a despairing attempt to recover the position and to improve the family's attitude. Of course it has the opposite effect. An employed man may keep a mounting portion of his income for 'pocket money' or, if they budget that way, his wife may discover that her monthly allowance has not been paid into her account. Even more distressing is when she finds out that payments for which he was responsible, hire purchase or building society instalments for instance, have not been made. He has been deceiving her. From her point of view she is forced to the recognition that he has been conducting a sort of family embezzlement. In hard terms there is less money available and *debts accumulate*. Similarly, this may happen to the husband of an alcoholic wife. The family has to live at a lower standard. Understandably there is all the more blame because the money has been squandered so pointlessly. At the same time the spouse begins to appreciate that they are *becoming isolated socially*. They get fewer invitations and the partner's state makes it advisable to refuse some of those still received. Increasingly the alcoholic's partner has to take over the full running of the family. Now the non-alcoholic partners organize, control and provide for everybody. They are increasingly driven to brood over the fact that their spouses have become inconsiderate, furtive and deceitful, seemingly callous and unfeeling. Added to which, they are often drunk. The alcoholic's manner becomes coarser. They are *repeatedly aggressive*, ill-treating their partner and abusing the children. At times they may hit. The result of such behaviour is a growing animosity towards them.

As the spouse accuses, rails, threatens and humiliates the other, the alcoholic retaliates with greater hostility. He or she is unable to see that all these adverse circumstances flow from his or her drinking. 'At first I compromised between marriage and drink. Then my home began to mean less. I spent increasing time in pubs and wanted more opportunities for drinking.' Alcoholics are led to re-interpret events in a paranoid way. We term this *the paranoid shift*. They see themselves as the victim, not as the originator, of the bad things that happen. It is their friends, employers or family who have let *them* down. Self-pity has come to partner their remorse.

This is also a point of no return. The opportunity for an important step in insight has been lost. Once alcoholics believe themselves wronged, they cease to construe the world correctly. They suspect those who try to help them, imagining them imbued with the hostility which they sense all around. Now, when coming home late they offer themselves a new reason for lingering in the pub. They used to feel remorse about this; now they persuade themselves that they are justified in doing so to escape from a nagging spouse's reproach. Similar *excuses and alibis* justify the opportunities found for drinking and the growing inability to meet responsibilities.

In fact, rationalizations began a long time ago, when the alcoholic first persuaded himself or herself that a drink might help in the way of business or social life. At first, it was persuading oneself; now one is persuaded, and it is a short step to being actually deluded. So, for instance, although it is *diminished sexual drive* which has made intercourse a rare occurrence, the male alcoholic comes to believe that this is the result of his wife's not wanting it. Her coldness provides him with the grain of truth needed to reinforce this notion. Then, suddenly, the idea will come to him that the reason for her unresponsiveness is that she has a lover. He is impervious to reassurance, to protestation; despite all evidence to the contrary he is convinced of her infidelity. He has become *morbidly jealous*, or she has in the case of a female alcoholic.

> I picture occasions my wife may have for intercourse. I become bitter, sick to my stomach, as if it's a lump of lead there. I feel I must do something more positive. I suspect the paternity of my second son. Then I wonder over the fact that the daughter coming after him also has red hair. I ask my wife would she permit a blood test. I feel low when I am accusing my wife but I have to see if I can break her down.

At about this time alcoholics may begin to be *continuously drunk throughout whole weekends*. Friday night to Sunday passes in a besotted blur. With the return of sobriety they may be able to remember very little of how the time has been passed. For the family, too, it has been a nightmare. If the alcoholic was at home and incapable then the family's contempt was excited; worse, if he or she did not come home, they had to reconcile their anger with their anxiety.

This state is not compatible with working properly at the beginning of the week. Missed days of work become more frequent, and eventually the alcoholic is out of a job. Either they get the sack or, realizing that this is inescapable, they quit. It is more difficult to find a second job than to keep the first one. A new employer will feel little compunction at dismissing them. And so it goes on. Forced into increasingly unskilled jobs for less and less money, alcoholics find themselves applying for posts which they would not have considered previously; and often they fail to get these.

The family may now break up. The alcoholic may leave home and go to live in lodgings fending for himself or herself. Isolated, they begin to look seedy and shabby, and people avoid them all the more. The last remnants of self-respect make them shun friends and they in turn keep out of the alcoholic's way.

When they wake up *in the morning they are restless* and anxious and find their hands are shaking. They cannot tie their shoe-laces, a man is not able to shave. Only if a drink is taken do the shakes come under control and dressing can be completed. *Morning drinking* now becomes a regular feature. Alcohol replaces a more orthodox breakfast for which the alcoholic has no stomach. The alcoholic guards against the possibility of being unable to moderate these symptoms by seeing to it that there are *always supplies of drink available*, if necessary by concealing bottles in every possible hiding-place. Sometimes they forget where they have put them and are beset with terror until they can remember.

A solicitor, still living with his wife, wrote this wry description:

The lavatory cistern's no use. Behind the pedestal of the wash hand basin in the bathroom is almost a common denominator. The high shelf in the linen cupboard is good enough because you are tall and the wife short. The rabbit hutch is undoubtedly in the clever class — rabbits can't talk; but too sudden an interest in animal life can give rise to disaster. The best of all is undoubtedly the car – that blanked-off bit in the dashboard where the radio used to be, underneath the tool kit, alongside the spare wheel, or just simply in the glove locker with last Sunday's newspaper on top of it. The decoy system has its merits, involving concealment in a place likely to give the hunter sufficient satisfaction in finding it that she will not want to look else-where. Perhaps the safest place of all is the inside jacket pocket, provided the tell-tale 'glug, glug' can be eliminated. Ability to remove and replace corks, stoppers, patent tops and the like quickly is another essential for the regular operator and demands constant practice and attention to detail. Nothing is more difficult to hide behind a screen of idle chatter than the all-pervading smell of whisky emanating from a leaking bottle.

At this stage alcoholics make strenuous attempts to stop, because they realize that drink is conquering them. They may at last be ready to concede that they are indeed alcoholics and that unless someone takes them in hand they are lost. With a mixture of determination and hopelessness they may manage on their own to abstain for a short while; generally these *dry periods* are measured in days only. Each spell is painfully achieved, for to begin it the physical and mental agony of withdrawal symptoms must be endured. One patient said:

> I realized I was drinking too much, and for about a year I managed to cut my input down; I restricted my drinking to weekends and drank mostly beer. But I gradually slipped back into the old pattern. Occasionally I tried to stop altogether but couldn't.

Sometimes there is an unfortunate accompaniment to these attempts to give up drinking. The alcoholic may seek to relieve the tension by *recourse to drugs* – tranquillizers, sleeping tablets or stimulants of the benzedrine group. The habit of taking these drugs is then likely to persist and is an additional serious complication. Moreover, the combination of drugs and alcohol may be very serious.

After each attempt to stop, drinking starts up again, and with it there is mounting dejection. Episodes of attempted suicide or self-injury which the alcoholic survives are frequent:

> I was dry for almost a month, but at my cousin's wedding I felt different from the others. I decided to have one drink. I thought I could control it. The old alcoholic delusion . . . I drank without restraint for the next five days. In a blinding flash of drunken logic I saw how bad I was. It was a shattering thunderbolt. I took a handful of pills, not as a cry for help but because of the hopeless position I was in.

Such episodes generally take place during a drinking spell, and the disturbance in thinking caused by intoxication distorts both the motive and the planning. Very often an overdose of pills is taken impulsively, without more than a moment's consideration. When such patients recover consciousness in hospital, they often cannot explain why they did it. Those who can may be unsure whether they intended to die or to force their plight upon people's notice. A man woke one morning to find himself sitting in his car in a park. He had had an amnesia. He had no idea how he got there. In a panic he drove to his home. His wife had left, taking all her belongings. He drank more, wrote a farewell letter to his wife and got into his car. 'I decided to crash in my car.' He drove at great speed into a lorry. He was taken to hospital unconscious with a fractured skull.

Underlying all these attempts is *despair*, sometimes arising suddenly after an evening's drinking, sometimes brooded over at length. Almost every alcoholic who has reached this degree of illness has ruminated that it would be better to be out of the way, better dead. As we have described in Chapter 3, many alcoholics kill themselves.

Chronic Alcoholism

The alcoholic is not eating enough now; he or she cannot be bothered to cook because the prolonged effect of alcohol on the stomach has taken the appetite away. Nausea is almost continuous. *Neglect of nutrition* may lead to physical illness, and this may give the doctor the first opportunity to discover the facts and confront the alcoholic with the diagnosis. The nutritional disorders that develop give rise to clear-cut physical disease.

We are now dealing with a chronic alcoholic, steeped in drink. The uninterrupted binges of intoxication, the prolonged periods of continuous drunkenness, are produced by less and less alcohol, for the body's *tolerance diminishes* quite sharply at this time. Alcoholics discover that they cannot drink anything like the quantity formerly consumed. The reduced intake no longer satisfies and, what is more, it produces disorganization and helplessness where previously there may have been pride about how much could be taken without getting drunk. Alcoholics always realize that this reduction in tolerance indicates a serious physical deterioration. Although binges are no longer pleasurable, they give themselves up to them. They *must have drink*, and to get it they will go to any lengths. They may start *drinking cheap wines*, even methylated spirits.

They become the *victims of terrifying fears*. Sometimes these accompany the drinking. Most of the time *thinking is confused*. Not to drink is torture, but drinking itself no longer brings relief. They may seek the help of Alcoholics Anonymous or go to a doctor for medical advice about alcoholism. Such advice may come, however, only upon admission to hospital with a *serious illness*, either a physical condition, usually cirrhosis of the liver or peripheral neuritis, or else with a psychiatric complication, delirium tremens, alcoholic epilepsy or a psychosis.

To continue drinking is now impossible; yet to stop is unthinkable. The chronic alcoholic admits defeat. He is on the road to death. If he is to live he must find treatment.

Chapter 9

The Alcoholic's Family

Just as alcoholics conform to definite types both in personality and in drinking pattern, so there are recognized patterns of behaviour in their spouses. Partly these are evolved as responses to the partner's drinking; we ought nevertheless to consider whether they might not have been present earlier. Most of what is known and written about the family of the alcoholic concern male alcoholics. This chapter is written principally from this aspect, but we shall later on refer to problems caused to the family by female alcoholics.

The Family of the Male Alcoholic

We should first consider whether male alcoholics select certain types of women and whether there are women who are particularly attracted to alcoholics, remembering that at the time of the marriage, alcoholism or even excessive drinking may not have developed. About half the spouses later to become alcoholic already drink excessively when they marry.[19] The women who accept them may be choosing their husbands because their personality characteristics appeal.

The wife of an alcoholic, much more frequently than chance would account for, is the daughter of an alcoholic. She may be seeking to revive in her marriage the relationship which she had with her father. Because she can see the justness of her friends' warnings, she may be hard put to account for her persistence in wanting to marry the man of her choice. She may marry him sensing full well that the marriage is not going to be happy. Her parents' objections are also no deterrent.

Male alcoholics frequently marry women older than themselves. This may perhaps indicate that the husband seeks maternal responses from his wife; he has created a psychological equivalent of his relationship with his mother. Some men who marry older women are sexually inhibited. They may tolerate, even welcome, being dominated by their wives who are the real authorities in the family. In the case of an alcoholic, this domination is frequently benign. His wife may enjoy mothering her husband, even when she has young children to nurture. She loves babies, wants many of them and may happily number her husband among them. Apart from isolated observations like these, information about wives of alcoholics is derived from questioning them after the alcoholism has developed. An alcoholic's wife often admits that she was aware that her husband drank a lot at the time she married him, but she will claim that she had not realized the implications of this. She expresses surprise, in retrospect, that she failed to do so. Many women, on the other hand, marry excessive drinkers believing that they will have a reforming influence upon their husbands. They do not realize how beset with conflict the marriage will be. From the wife's standpoint, her husband will not be dependable; she will have to manage the greater part of the household responsibilities on her own. She cannot rely on him to play his part either in important decisions or in day-to-day choices. There may be prolonged periods during which he is unemployed and she is the breadwinner. Any assistance he then renders takes the form of domestic duties, cooking, cleaning and childminding.

She becomes insensitive to the effect on him of her constantly disparaging and belittling reaction. One wife, genuinely anxious to be helpful to her husband, described in detail his 'dim-witted behaviour'. She dwelt with careful emphasis on his social clumsiness.

He tries desperately hard. He wants to be extra nice. He says unusual things, like 'What a nice hat' – you know – without realizing sufficiently that what he is saying is unusual. When there is talk about business, he makes remarks which have an air of wisdom but nothing behind them. When people ask him a question about his work or something factual the answer he gives is perfectly futile, even to an outsider. I feel that anyone would know it was a guess. In conversation with me, and particularly when we have other people around, he will make statements about matters of which he knows nothing. They are totally incorrect, and he can't substantiate them. He tries to if discussion arises, not really aggressively but . . . he feels he has to assert himself. He makes the mistake of thinking that what matters is asserting himself and is not sure if he is right when he does so.

More than one writer has stressed how capable an alcoholic's wife often is. She can generally manage the household affairs on her own and, to the outsider at least, she seems to have no great need for an adequate husband. Towards her children she feels competent to combine the father's role with her own. And by assuming this complete parental function she diminishes her husband in his own eyes, thus underlining his sense of inadequacy.

Because those who treat the male alcoholic must have him as their primary focus of concern, they may view the wife as a determining or at least an aggravating factor in her husband's condition. Because they must mobilize every resource towards improving his state they are apt to concentrate on those facets of the wife's behaviour which may exacerbate his drinking. Many wives consider that their husbands are getting more attention than they deserve, whilst they themselves are neglected by the helpers. When their husbands are receiving treatment, some wives feel that the treatment staff are inferring that they are somehow to blame for their husband's condition. If either party merits criticism, the wife considers it is surely the offending husband because of the way he has treated her. An alcoholic can make things very hard for his wife. At the most material level, he is spending far too much of their money, and she knows where it is all going. When she protests, he may make promises, but matters always get worse. How could they improve when he is compelled to spend upwards of £40 a week on drink? It costs more than that for half a bottle of whisky a day even if you drink at home. Try as she may, the wife cannot maintain the home standards she wishes and feels that she justly deserves. Debts mount but her husband appears unconcerned: when she plans to economize she gets no support from her husband.

Socially, too, he is no longer dependable. She never knows when he will be home for meals, and if she prepares food it may be wasted. She cannot arrange for them to go out to friends for he may not be willing. She dare not invite friends home for he may not be sober. In short she cannot plan, so no coherent way of life is possible for her. Alcoholics' wives wait. They wait for their husbands to come home; they wait for an accident; they wait for their husbands to lose their jobs. They wait for the inevitable catastrophe.

The wife witnesses his intoxicated behaviour, day after day, week after week, with increasing abhorrence. He himself is only partly aware of what he is doing. It is she who sees how appalling some of his actions are. At times he seems blatantly loutish and brutish to her. Mostly she feels that he is incapable of decent behaviour. His behaviour always hurts, whether she regards this as intentional on his part or not. She sees him insidiously and progressively destroying all she had come to hope for and to expect from life. She may have to endure his violence; by no means all alcoholics are violent when intoxicated, but many can be. He may be jealous and accuse her of going with other men. She can be severely ill-treated, both physically and mentally. This quarrelling, rowing and violence is inevitably a great strain on the family.

His sexual approaches may repel her by their unfeeling clumsiness. What had been of emotional importance is so no longer. Fear of becoming pregnant when her husband is in such a state increases her distaste for intercourse, which seems to her to be degrading, merely a satisfying of his transient and ineffective lust.

There are no signs of companionship, warmth or understanding from the husband. There is no opportunity for them to talk together, so she cannot convey to him her own thoughts and experiences and needs. Even where she is able to, she questions whether he would understand, appreciate and respond. She feels herself increasingly solitary, her life arid from the lack of affection and the impossibility of expressing tenderness towards him.

A wife may lavish her uninvested emotion on the children, swamping them with excessive demands to make good the deficit in her marriage and to provide the affection which she does not get from her husband. Children are not mature enough to meet these emotional pressures, and their own development can be harmed by the pressures upon them to do so.

The alcoholic's wife is bewildered and unable to put into perspective what has happened in her life. She ponders whether she has brought it upon herself. She fears at times that she may be responsible for her husband's drinking. She cannot decide if he is unfeeling, wilful or sick. She does not know if it is more appropriate for her to be angry or protective. She does not know what view to take of the problem or to whom to turn for help. She may continue for a long time, vainly hoping that her husband is just going through a bad patch, that the upset is only temporary, and that by his own efforts he will yet manage to control his drinking.

She spends a lot of her energy covering up for him. She dissembles to his employers about his lateness, his absences or his early departures from work. She parries neighbours' puzzled inquiries or unwanted expressions of sympathy. She attempts, with less success than she knows, to conceal from her children the slights to which she is subjected and the quarrels which ensue. Her parents begin urging her to take a strong line with him, even to leave him, and she is in conflict between her filial and her marital loyalties.

The wife tries what have been called 'home remedies', the vain devices aimed at removing available liquor. Bottles are searched for, emptied down the sink, hidden; attempts are made to control the money, to persuade shops not to allow credit. Decisions are made, promises extracted, ultimatums delivered. The wife persists in the hopeless sequence of pleading, argument, hostility, hatred, because she does not grasp yet that, much as her husband would wish to stop drinking, only with specialized outside assistance will he be able to give up alcohol. In the meantime, the family may live through quarrels, terror, physical assault and neighbourhood disgrace. The wife may be unable to tolerate more distress, or she may decide that for the sake of the children she has to leave her husband.

If she can only come to understand that what besets her husband is illness, a new way of dealing with problems opens for her. She can cease to hold her husband wilfully responsible for what he is doing to her, and her natural affection and sympathies for him need no longer be withheld.

A patient's wife was telling the doctor about his behaviour when drinking, alternately talking to the doctor and rounding on her husband who was present:

Once he starts drinking nothing you can say makes sense to him. There's an imbecilic look on his face. You're just not in the same world at all. It's a completely different person! He talks rubbish. Everything makes him quarrelsome. You get the failings of everybody thrown at you all the time. I don't think you even remember what happens, or all the things you say. An objectionable, horrible person, completely different. Such a horrible creature. It's a terrible Jekyll and Hyde thing. It's as if he takes a blackout or a brainstorm. It's not that he's drunk: all sense seems to go completely out.

It's difficult to move him from one room to another. You try to make him go into the bedroom, to get him out of sight. He fights you. You try to stop him from damaging himself when swaying too violently. You can't reason with him – I'm told I'm completely useless, quite hopeless, I'm told I can't face life as it really is. I find bottles about the room and tell him. He says, 'There were no bottles in the room.' He tells me he has stopped, and I find one bottle in the bed and one under the car seat. Then he drinks champagne to celebrate finishing with drink for all time. You really have to live with it to know what it's like. My goodness, I can sympathize with any wife who goes through this. Now I've got to think of the boys – my one son is disgusted with his father; the other won't go near him.

When the wife stopped speaking her husband glared at her and said quietly: 'What you really want to see happen is that I should be locked up.' His wife did not deny the hostility she had been driven to feel. She said helplessly, 'If I stopped seeing it as an illness that would be hopeless. If I thought he could help it, that would be the end.'

The wife who has learnt to regard her husband's alcoholism as an illness can go on to orient her own life with greater assurance, even if her husband should continue to drink. As far as her feelings are concerned she may still oscillate between sympathy and anger. But she no longer has to feel ineffectual, overwhelmed by the problem. She can now approach the resources in society that can provide help. Professional people are becoming increasingly enlightened about the problem of alcoholism, and the misguided attitudes of previous times are giving way to better counsels today. So the doctor, the minister, the lawyer or the social worker need not nowadays limit their advice to moralizing. The doctor or alcohol treatment agency can advise on a suitable course of action and inform the wife what treatment will be available. She may be recommended to adopt a certain approach if her husband is cooperative, but if he is not she can still be helped to decide what to do. There are few doctors today who will tell the wife that her alcoholic husband is worthless, urging her to leave him. Ministers can offer practical advice to suit the particular need in addition to the prayer and faith which they have always advocated. Social workers no longer dispense ready-made drastic advice or solutions, but investigate with the spouse the special circumstances of the case. Should a wife want to stay with her husband, this will be appreciated by members of these helping professions. If she is determined to leave him, they will not criticize. If she cannot make up her mind, they will not make the decision for her but will assist her in weighing up the merits of each course. A decision on her part to separate may not be the drastic undoing of her husband that she fears. The fact of, or threat of, a wife's leaving may make an alcoholic more prepared to go for treatment. An excess of care by a supportive wife, especially if the dependent relationship shields the alcoholic from what would otherwise be the realities of his condition, may actually militate against his acceptance of treatment.

The involvement of family members in the treatment of the alcoholic has become standard practice in many programmes.[20] The more cohesive a marriage the better the outcome; the quality of interaction in the marriage is one of the best predictors of outcome.[21]

Marriages of alcoholics are often interrupted by separations and many end in divorce. Either the alcoholic or the spouse may initiate the separation but it is usually the latter, because the alcoholic has much more to lose than to gain by leaving home. If we are considering male alcoholics it is generally late in the progress of the condition that they quit the home, and often it is the wife who brings this about, not the alcoholic. Sometimes the wife leaves, taking the children with her and retreating to her mother's house or to another member of the family. She does it because she can no longer stand the drunken behaviour at home and the humiliation of never being able to go out or to have friends call; she does it to protect her children from the repugnant sight of their father and, last but not least, she does it to exert pressure on him to stop drinking or to go for treatment. These separations may not last long; the wife yields to his pleas for her return and his protestations that he will reform. When next he relapses it will be less of a struggle for her to leave. So there are often a number of separations. By themselves these do not necessarily indicate that the marriage will end. It is considerably more likely to do so when the husband has lost his job or has been physically violent to his family. Then his wife often concludes that the marriage is hopeless and makes a decision never to return. Whether or not such a final separation is taken to the divorce courts depends on many extraneous factors.

When the wife remains with her husband she may none the less harbour intensely painful feelings of resentment and anger towards him. She is sometimes not fully aware of this hostility. Though she does not voice it directly she can use others in the family to give expression to it.

One alcoholic gave up drink when treated and, after leaving hospital, returned to work and regularly attended the weekly outpatient psychotherapeutic group, in which he was exploring the problems that he had in relationships with others.

His wife's father, who lived in the house with them, was an irritation to the patient. The old man would rarely leave the house: he was involved in all the family discussions, recalling how difficult the alcoholic had been, the hardships his daughter had suffered, the disadvantages inflicted on the children, and so on. When the patient had a temporary lapse he was ashamed and dejected. To his wife's reproaches were added the old man's portentous predictions of imminent disaster: everything was hopeless, all was now lost. The alcoholic drank more, grabbed sleeping pills from the medicine cupboard and swallowed a large number in the presence of his wife and father-in-law. He sat down and gradually got drowsy. As he became unconscious, the father urged: 'Leave him.' It was only when the 12-year-old son returned home that the mother was persuaded to call the doctor, who then summoned an ambulance to convey the by now unconscious man to hospital.

There are marriages in which the wife of the alcoholic herself becomes ill. Her illness may be bodily or psychological. One of our patients, after her criminal and drunken alcoholic husband had abused and hit her and gone out, and her two teenaged daughters had unsympathetically advised her to bolt the door against his return, and had then themselves gone out, sat down and wept. 'And then I thought, "Sod the lot of them" and went upstairs and took all my tablets.' What she clearly thought was that everyone else was selfishly going their own way and no one seemed to want to help her. She was right.

Sometimes the wife's illness, paradoxically, only starts when the husband stops drinking, the first symptoms appearing when he assumes increasing family responsibility. When this occurs it is a serious added strain to the husband, often jeopardizing his recovery. Fortunately it is not common. One alcoholic had recovered satisfactorily with treatment and resumed his part in his family's affairs. An unmarried daughter had become pregnant, and when the time came for her delivery she was living in a distant city with a married sister. The recovered patient wanted to go with his wife on the visit she had planned to support her daughter through this difficult time. He intended to urge his daughter to end her association with the man responsible for the pregnancy. He succeeded in conveying his point of view, but his wife became involved in a quarrel with the married daughter whose house it was. As a result, she was told to leave. Thereupon she lost her memory, and for months afterwards was disabled by a psychological disorder of fluctuating severity, in which she was unable to recall how many children she had and how old they were; at times she was even uncertain whether she was married or not.

Notwithstanding the great stresses imposed, most wives stay with their husbands through painful years of disappointment, debt and humiliation; they assist them energetically to obtain treatment, seek advice themselves to understand how they might have contributed to their husbands' difficulty, and are profoundly happy with the contentment and order which results when their husbands' drinking stops.

The Family of the Female Alcoholic

When the wife is alcoholic increased burdens fall on the husband and upon the older children. There can be one important difference: the husband has a semblance of a normal social life when out of the home at work. Only in the evenings, when he may be tired, does he have to face the shambles of his home and the tirades that fill the hours before he can go to bed. Many husbands, just as we have seen is done by many wives, put up with such a life for a considerable time, particularly in middle-class families. The husband gets the children off to school, keeps the house as clean as he may, does the shopping and cooks the meals, unless the children are capable. Very often a close cohesive relationship develops between father and children in these circumstances, designed both to cover up the situation from neighbours and to provide mutual support. Husbands whose whole attitude to their wives is hostile and recriminating tend not to stay, so the treatment agency that finds a situation where the husband is still living with his alcoholic wife can usually count on his support.

On the other hand, such husbands rarely accept that anything they might have done, or not done, any animosity or lack of affection from them, can have played any part in determining their wives' alcoholism. As a consequence they are more reluctant than are wives of alcoholic men to feel the need to be involved in discussions to understand better the reasons for their wives' drinking.

Children of Alcoholics

Possible genetic effects of an alcoholic parent have been considered in Chapter 6; here we are concerned only with the familial effects of alcoholism.

A competent mother can make up for most of the deficiencies resulting from a father's alcoholism. So pronounced are the capabilities of alcoholics' wives to sustain the roles proper to their husbands that the children do not commonly suffer material privation. Inevitably the personal development of the children of an alcoholic must be anomalous, but this need not give rise to any adult disorder. They are certain to have a decided attitude towards drinkers and drinking, either tending to drink excessively themselves or becoming strongly opposed to it. Sons of alcoholics frequently become alcoholic themselves. Their personalities have been labelled 'passive-aggressive';[22] they often have serious difficulty in expressing assertive impulses and in knowing what to do with angry feelings aroused by frustrating situations. Male alcoholics often stress that they have perceived their drinking fathers as nebulous family members, inaccessible when their presence was longed for. These sons envied other boys who were proud of fathers that took an interest in their achievements and played with them.

The alcoholic father is often as good as absent, always liable to erupt unpredictably with behaviour that embarrasses or wounds the family. The children quickly pick up cues from their mother, leading them to look down on their father and condemn his standards and actions. A son of such a father never loses the impact made on him by the paternal failure. One alcoholic would never enter a hotel; he could not bring himself to do so, being constrained by recollections of repeated humiliations during his adolescence caused by his father's uncouth and uninhibited behaviour to waitresses. He felt himself enfeebled and deprived through never having had a father who could be respected.

The effect of an alcoholic parent persists throughout life; its influence is subtle and strong. Attitudes are conditioned by it, whether or not the individual is aware of this. We have seen that a girl whose father was an alcoholic will often marry a passive man, perhaps even an alcoholic himself. She may repeat the same pattern two or three times. An alcoholic father provides an unserviceable personality model.

In Sweden children of alcoholic fathers were compared with similar children from non-alcoholic families.[23] The ages ranged from four to twelve years. Divorce or separation had taken place in 28 per cent of the alcoholic families and in 4 per cent of the control families. One of the comparisons made was in attendances at hospital: 24 per cent from the alcoholics' families, and a similar figure, 19 per cent, from the controls', had been to hospital. But whereas two thirds of the control children had organic causes found to account for their physical symptoms, this was true for only a quarter of the alcoholics' children. Attendances at child-guidance clinics, for psychiatric disorder, were the same for the two groups of children. When their teachers were questioned they rated 48 per cent of children from alcoholic families as problem children, but only 10 per cent of those from non-alcoholic homes. In another investigation also cited previously,[24] children of alcoholics (not known to be so by their teachers) were regarded by them less favourably than children randomly picked for comparison from the same class.

Tension in the child shows not only in the form of illnesses and abnormal behaviour at school but also in disturbed relationships at home.

Children of alcoholics are particularly likely to have conduct or behaviour disorders. In one investigation the children of alcoholics were characterized by temper tantrums, destructive behaviour and hyperactivity.[25] These symptoms were more frequent in the families where violence had been prominent. Children of alcoholics have been found to have special difficulty in making friends.[26] They are, as we have mentioned, at risk of alcoholism themselves when adult.

Where the father is alcoholic, an intensified relationship is set up between the children and their mother; she may thus unwittingly become the recipient of hostile and resentful feelings which the total family situation has engendered in the children. In carrying out the breadwinning role on her own, the mother had perforce to neglect some of her other functions. Nylander found that the alcoholics' children who had had to be admitted to hospital for psychiatric care seemed to have more problems concerning their mothers than their fathers.

The effect upon the child of an alcoholic parent is considerably reduced if the other parent is able to provide a sympathetic explanation of the condition in terms of illness. This enables the child to understand why a father fails so grossly in his paternal role, or an alcoholic woman in her maternal role, and so spares the growing child some of the harmful effects which result when a parent is viewed with contempt. There can be no doubt that where a parent is known to be alcoholic, the entire family is under strain and at risk, and help is needed to alleviate the stress of family members over and above the care given to the alcoholic. We ought not, however, to leave an impression that the children of alcoholics inevitably fare badly. The effects of having an alcoholic parent do, as we have stated, persist throughout life; nevertheless most children of alcoholics overcome these difficulties and make an adequate adjustment.

Chapter 10

Treatment

General Considerations

Treatment of an alcoholic is a large endeavour. It is not, however, a complicated matter. A myth has arisen that it is so difficult that it can only be carried out by experts, whether doctors or those belonging to other health professions, or else by specialist self-help organizations such as Alcoholics Anonymous. It is true that some alcoholics, because of their special physical, psychological or social circumstances, do require expert services; however, the majority of alcoholics can be successfully treated by staff who are willing to give the time, concern and interest to alcoholics and have the determination to see the treatment through, even though they may not have had special training in the subject. Nor is it necessary for the alcoholic to be sent anywhere special for treatment. Only a small minority need to be admitted to a special facility for their treatment. Within the context of medicine, therefore, it is perfectly possible for general physicians or general practitioners to treat their alcoholic patients; similarly, social workers, nurses and clinical psychologists, subject to what we shall say later about the need for medical examination, can treat alcoholics satisfactorily and successfully. The mythology that only by getting to an expert in alcoholism can an alcoholic be helped is damaging. It is not the case, and just as well, because specialist services are only available in sufficient extent to deal with the difficult problems to which we have referred.

Before treatment can begin there first has to be recognition that the condition exists and, second, the individual has to be persuaded that treatment is available and that he or she needs it.

Almost invariably, alcoholics have recognized their problem for themselves, although they may not have wished to do so. They may strenuously deny it when others challenge them about it (though often this comes as a relief), but there are few alcoholics who are not aware both that they are drinking excessively and that it is doing them harm. They shrink from the word *alcoholic*, but they accept the problem.

In this they may be well ahead of their medical advisers. We believe that other professionals, social workers, probation officers, nurses, health visitors, psychologists, who come up against alcoholism in their clients, may also fail in the task of recognition, but our information is principally about members of the medical profession.

The average-sized general practice will contain about thirty alcoholics. Only a tenth of them are recognized as such by their doctors, although they are known as sick individuals.[27] Owens[28] studied random admissions to male medical wards in the four principal general hospitals in Manchester. He inquired in a detailed way into both drinking and harms. According to his criteria, 18 per cent of these admissions were alcoholics, and in two thirds of cases alcohol could be implicated in the aetiology of their medical illness. Gastroenterological disease and drug overdose were the principal clinical disorders. The medical staff were aware of the alcoholism in only half of these patients, and when they did know, it was frequently not clinical acumen but the patient's history of treatment for the condition that was the indicator.

Jariwalla and his co-workers[29] reported a study conducted in the Manchester Royal Infirmary which more than supports Owens's work, as do Jarman and Kellett.[30] In 27 per cent of admissions to acute medical beds, alcohol was considered to be a relevant factor, and this was so for 16 per cent of patients with physical illness, i.e. excluding overdoses. Is there any other medical condition so frequent in its occurrence, so serious in its consequences, and so potentially susceptible to treatment, that physicians fail to diagnose half the times they should?

Doctors need to recognize alcoholism and should learn how to detect it. They should know how to elicit a history of drinking and how to inquire into the harms of alcohol. Detection is best done clinically, yet Barrison *et al.*[31] discovered that doctors did not take drinking histories from patients even when their medical knowledge surely indicated the need. It will be a relief to clinicians to learn that their diagnostic difficulties can be overcome by easily learned clinical skills. Yet at a conference held in 1986 by the Department of Health,[32] five newly appointed independent medical specialists (a general practitioner, a community physician and three hospital consultants, including a psychiatrist) each said that they had received next to no education about alcohol during their postgraduate training, and in consequence had, on appointment, felt inadequate in coping with alcoholics. They learned subsequently. There remain important educational tasks for doctors and probably for members of other professional groups.

One reason why alcoholism is not detected is that doctors may not wish to engage in a discussion which they fear will come close to criticism of their patients. Yet it is their duty and must not be avoided. The same applies to the other professionals we have mentioned, and it applies, moreover, to employers, personnel managers, friends and family members. It is the first step in persuading the alcoholic to accept treatment.

Sometimes it is right to apply a degree of pressure. This may take the form of spelling out the medical or social consequences, but the most important element in the persuasion is to point out to the alcoholic that help is available, telling him or her exactly how and where it can be arranged and also that treatment can be effective. Another very positive feature in the persuasion is letting the alcoholic know that you are not being judgemental but supportive and that the support will continue.

The Treatment Plan

The first element in treatment is the formulation of a treatment plan, which needs to be based on an agreed objective for the treatment. The plan and the objective must be tailor-made to suit the circumstances of the patient. Over and over again the reason for treatment failure turns out to be failure to agree upon an objective. For instance, alcoholism treatment units like to try to induce their patients to become abstinent. This may be appropriate for many alcoholics, yet for those in its advanced stages, with body and brain damage and an incapacity to work, the appropriate objective may be just to prevent further deterioration and to secure a roof over their heads. They need provision of food and shelter much more than help to stop drinking. They are not going to stop drinking. All too often we have observed the development of a stand-off position where the doctor, say, asks the alcoholic to enter a regime of treatment designed to produce abstinence and then accuses the alcoholic (that is often how it seems) of unwillingness to cooperate. It is a small step then to the alcoholic being rejected for treatment. Those treating alcoholics must be flexible in their objectives and discuss these with their patients so that there can be agreement on what both are striving for. Achieving agreement about the objective of treatment puts one half-way on the road to success. The alcoholic patient should not be simply told 'This is the programme we offer', and then blamed for being unprepared or unwilling to conform to it. We may conclude this introductory statement by saying that all those in the team that undertakes the treatment should be working to a common purpose, and that includes the patient.

The formulation of an objective of treatment and of the plan to effect it requires a thorough assessment of the situation. This involves taking a detailed drinking history and knowing what consequences of alcoholism the patient has undergone. The assessment needs to take into account what led to the excessive drinking and the alcoholic's present life circumstances. These include the extent of his or her social supports, the financial position, and the physical and mental state. There must, therefore, be a detailed medical examination including a psychological examination. For this reason we insist that although people other than doctors can be appropriate to treat alcoholics, they should not embark upon treatment until a doctor has examined the patient, carrying out medical and psychological investigations if necessary, and come to a conclusion about his medical state. Once this has been done it may well be safe for the alcoholic's treatment to be carried out by non-medical people. This rule applies to alcoholics at whatever stage they may be.

Neglect of a medical examination is a dereliction of care. Other information that has to be gathered concerns past illnesses, physical and mental, the history of the family and any past attempts to stop or limit drinking, whether spontaneously or as a result of treatment.

It has to be borne in mind when devising the treatment programme that drinking may be the only way the alcoholic has found to deal with life's problems. Alcoholics usually very well know the harm that alcohol is doing to them but feel that without it they cannot cope. If this is the case then it will not be sufficient merely to wean them from alcohol, since when they must once again face their problems they will be bereft of any means except to revert again to the bottle. So, to restrict treatment merely to depriving the alcoholic of alcohol is not enough. Alcoholics need to be supported so that they can deal with their problems in a better fashion, and an attempt must also be made to reduce the problems, if at all possible. Indeed we should go further and strengthen the alcoholics so that they master their problems without support, at any rate without continually having to rely upon treatment; support from family and friends may well, of course, be a constant resource for them.

Now we begin to see the strength of the man–problem–device model of cause that we have already considered. Any or all of these three elements may have to be addressed in a comprehensive treatment programme.

Withdrawing Alcohol – Detoxification

The device, the alcohol itself, is the easiest to tackle. Even if the patient is physically dependent on alcohol it is a relatively simple matter to effect alcohol withdrawal, a process which is currently called *detoxification*. Many patients go through it without experiencing any of the serious withdrawal effects we have described, and if they do occur they are usually limited to 'the shakes'. Medication is not always required, either as treatment or as prophylaxis. However, if the patient has had withdrawal symptoms previously, or they arise and are distressing, then medication can promptly and effectively suppress them. Tranquillizers are used, for short periods only. Commonly employed are a minor tranquillizer such as chlordiazepoxide (Librium) or a major tranquillizer: chlormethiazole (Heminevrin) is most used because it carries least risk of damage to the liver. Medications can be taken by mouth but, if there is urgency, it is possible to administer them by injection. Usually the detoxification process is over in one to five days; however, if it is necessary to suppress serious withdrawal symptoms then these medicines may have to be continued for up to a fortnight.

It used to be thought that every long-standing alcoholic was so likely to develop distressing withdrawal symptoms that medication to suppress them should routinely be given to cover withdrawal. However, one of the findings gained from the work of detoxification centres is that most alcoholics can readily manage without medication.[33] Nevertheless, because withdrawal symptoms may be unpleasant there is no justification for withholding medication if it is needed.

Detoxification deals with the immediate elimination of alcohol from the body, often coinciding with the onset of treatment. The principles of detoxification will be dealt with later in this chapter when we describe detoxification centres. Most alcoholics, however, detoxify themselves in their own homes. Alternatively it may take place in general hospitals or in psychiatric units.

Preventing Drinking Beginning Again

Antabuse (disulfiram) and Abstem (citrated calcium carbimide) may sometimes be given to patients who are no longer drinking to reduce the likelihood of their beginning to drink again. Each is taken in tablet form. These two preparations are chemically different, but in the body they act in identical ways. The objective is to make the experience of drinking alcohol unpleasant, which they do by interfering with the way the body deals with the alcohol. When alcohol is metabolized it is changed into carbon dioxide and water. At an intermediate stage in this chemical process a toxic substance, acetaldehyde, is formed, but it is so rapidly broken down that no ill effects are felt. The action of Antabuse or Abstem is to slow the breakdown of acetaldehyde so that when a person drinks, the level in the blood rises. The accumulating acetaldehyde brings about a sequence of physical sensations which each patient learns for himself.

The first symptom to occur in the Antabuse–alcohol reaction is flushing and warmth of the face. Then a pounding is felt at the temples as the heartbeat accelerates. A headache commonly develops. Another common effect is a catch in the breath, as if there is some sort of obstruction in the windpipe; there may be coughing or a choking sensation. The patient becomes uncomfortably aware of his breathing because he has to work harder to take in the necessary air. Anxiety generally accompanies the reaction, which is probably a direct effect of the acetaldehyde in the circulation.

Patients learn what their particular response is through a test reaction given by the doctor. Nobody should ever take Antabuse without having undergone such a test. Its purposes are twofold: to teach patients what to expect and to enable the doctor to cut the reaction short if it is unduly severe. The test takes the following form. Patients take a tablet each morning for at least three days and are then given two or four ounces of spirits or an equivalent amount of their usual drink. The reaction begins about ten minutes after taking the alcohol and lasts about an hour. It is very seldom distressing, but if so it can promptly be cut short. If the reaction to the test is so severe that this is necessary, then it is not wise to continue with either Antabuse or Abstem. The aim of the test is not to terrify the person taking it (this is in no way an 'aversion' treatment), but to let him or her learn from personal experience about how to use Antabuse to stop drinking. Once the test has been satisfactorily completed, patients routinely take a tablet every day. Thus they prevent themselves from drinking by the knowledge that alcohol will no longer achieve its pleasurable effect.

The effects of Antabuse occur if alcohol is taken within about three days of a tablet being taken. Once this period has elapsed, and the drug has been totally excreted from the system, no further adverse reactions will occur with drinking. The treatment works best if the tablet is taken at the same time each day, thus establishing the routine. The morning is best, because temptation to drink is often least at that time. The container should have its unvarying place with the toothbrush or on the breakfast table, so that the tablet may thus be taken without deliberation or inner debate. It is often helpful if the spouse participates sympathetically in the daily round of the tablet-taking. To those who protest against placing reliance on a pill rather than on will-power, alcoholics who have found Antabuse a worthy aid reply that they use their will-power to remember to take the tablet every morning.

Most helped by Antabuse or Abstem are those alcoholics who continue to experience strong cravings for alcohol for many months after becoming abstinent. They emphasize, eloquently, that they regularly want a drink very badly indeed. For them Antabuse or Abstem provides a sort of chemical security. The value to abstinent alcoholics of an Antabuse regime is that if a crisis should occur, which they are tempted to resolve through drinking, they cannot do so without waiting for three days until the drug has been eliminated from the body. By then the crisis may be over, or they may have taken adequate steps to deal with it, and so decide to resume the tablet-taking instead of the drinking. In the early stages of treatment, patients may rely heavily on Antabuse, because they can scarcely believe that it will prove possible for them to remain abstinent by their own efforts. They feel they cannot make the undertaking never to use alcohol again, and so they are reassured by the knowledge that, temporarily at any rate, it is impossible for them to drink. Paradoxically, in the case of those who continue to face life problems still seemingly insoluble, the knowledge that they have only to leave off Antabuse for three days, and then can drink again should such relief become imperative, is reassuring.

Occasionally, Antabuse or Abstem, even if the patient does not drink, may produce mildly unpleasant effects in certain individuals who are hypersensitive. The commonest is a metallic taste in the mouth, but others include skin rashes, a state of lethargy, headache, stomach discomfort and, rarely, a confusional episode. Such reactions, although infrequent, are another reason why the drug should only be used under experienced medical supervision. It is worthwhile, in such cases, to try Abstem if Antabuse has been used, or vice versa. Experience with long-acting implants of Antabuse has been very negative.

Antabuse or Abstem, correctly used, reduces the likelihood of impulsive drinking. However, they make up no more than a part of a comprehensive treatment programme; yet for some patients they may be life-saving. These people consider that only the daily tablet, the 'Antabuse habit', stands between their present sobriety and the resumption of uncontrolled drinking. Having taken the tablet, they have made their decision for that day. At a time when temptation is lowest they have thus protected themselves against craving that might arise later on, for instance from the otherwise overwhelming attraction of the smell that wafts towards them from an open public house door as they pass along the street.

No general answer can be given to how long the automatic taking of Antabuse should continue. The decision is best made jointly by patient and doctor. Some give up the tablets soon and stay well. It is probably unwise to give it up in under six months, and some patients comfortably continue for life. Often discussion makes it clear that the patient considers stopping Antabuse at a time of particular strain, such as trouble at work or disturbance in a personal relationship. Of course, this is just the time not to stop. It is important to make sure that a patient's decision to do without does not coincide with them turning over in their mind the possibility that they might consider returning to social drinking. Of course they are entitled to try this, but it needs full discussion with the doctor so that they understand how slim are the chances.

There is no justification for supposing that only the weak require Antabuse, and that to use it is to rely on a crutch. Each patient's alcoholism is an individual matter. Some alcoholics who choose to rely on Antabuse are among the most resolute of the patients we have known. They view Antabuse as an important medical discovery (they only wish that a drug was also discovered which could reduce the discomfort of craving). They use the analogy that if one were entering a malarial country one would take prophylactic medication. For them, going about the streets is to venture into dangerous territory.

Because Antabuse may be bought over the counter of a chemist's shop, three warnings should be given. It is unwise, and may be extremely dangerous, to start taking Antabuse without having been physically examined and without having had a trial reaction watched by a doctor. After having had some drinks it is unsafe to take Antabuse until the alcohol has been eliminated from the body; generally this means waiting twenty-four hours after the last drink. Finally the alcoholic has to know that he or she is on tablets; to do as some have done and give Antabuse to someone surreptitiously is not only misguided but dangerous. Under no circumstances should anyone, alcoholic or not, be given Antabuse without being told.

Social Work

By the time most alcoholics are ready to accept help, they are usually in some sort of social predicament, in connection with their family and friends, with their work, with the law, with debts, etc. The vicious-circle models we have used show that the more the drinking the worse the predicament, and also that the worse the predicament the more the patient may be driven to drink. Active intervention is often needed to break this circle. The problems appear overwhelming to alcoholics. They see no way out of them. The first thing to do is to arrange these problems in some order of priority: which are the most pressing, and which can wait. If alcoholics are helped to tackle them one by one, the task may start to seem worth undertaking. Then it is often possible to effect an amelioration. Debtors can be induced not to be so insistent and spouses to be less censorious and more supportive. This requires someone talking to the spouse and explaining how matters stand. At such a meeting it is important to appreciate the difficulties that the spouse has, but also to explain the predicament from the point of view of the alcoholic. The suffering spouse may not have been able to grasp that the alcoholic is suffering too and not just giving way to self-indulgence. Above all, the spouse needs to learn that he or she can be useful, a positive, indeed an essential, help in getting the alcoholic back on an even keel. Similarly it may be necessary to approach the police or the magistracy, usually via the probation service. Generally, provided no serious offence has been committed, the law is glad to learn that a treatment agency is involved and attempting to take charge of the situation. Both the police and the courts know that neither fines nor imprisonment benefit the situation. If the alcoholic's employment is threatened it may be helpful, though only with the patient's permission, to approach the employer or the personnel officer, to assure him or her that something is being done and to try to stabilize the situation.

Effecting these most essential steps is within the competence of a social worker, who may, if necessary, approach people directly on the patient's behalf but equally may try to persuade him or her, with help, to do as much as possible himself or herself. The social worker's intervention with the spouse also is crucial in treatment.

The Patient

The final part of the treatment triad is to work on the patients themselves. The simplest aspect of this consists in attending to any physical disabilities that may be present. Such treatment is squarely a medical responsibility. It involves consideration of patients' general nutrition and replacement of any vitamins lacking. There may have to be correction of anaemia and treatment of specific illnesses of the nervous system (including the brain), the liver, the stomach and the heart. These are the parts of the body principally affected. Unfortunately, it is not always possible to restore each of these organs to their healthy state. Almost always it cannot be done unless the patients stop drinking, and this may be particularly hard for them when physical disease has supervened.

To effect changes in patients' personalities, so that they become strengthened in their ability to deal with social problems or to overcome psychological illnesses that have occurred in the setting of their alcoholism, is the most complex part of treatment. Yet even this process should not be thought of as so difficult that it can only be done by experts. The principles underlying treatment are, first, to be accepting and totally non-judgemental; second, to encourage the alcoholics to discuss their problems, anxieties and fears fully and to look, if necessary critically, at their own behaviour; third, to let them view themselves as people not despicable and worthless, but of value both to themselves and to others, to foster in them a degree of self-respect; and last, to offer help for as long as the patients need it. Each of these is necessary and each demands of the helper that conjunction of dispassionate and compassionate skill and competence that betokens professionalism.

Psychotherapy

This kind of treatment, involving discussion between patient and therapist (of whatever professional background) is called *psychotherapy*. It makes demands on both the therapist's time and emotions. It calls for an evenness of approach, being neither critical in any way nor overly sympathetic. Such an approach, however, should be part of the therapeutic resource of all doctors, social workers and nurses, especially those whose work involves the treatment of alcoholics. Special psychotherapeutic techniques, such as behaviour therapy to correct faulty conditioning and maladaptive learning, may be offered by clinical psychologists; where alcoholism is secondary to psychoneurosis or personality disorder then psychoanalysis or other forms of intensive insight psychotherapy may be called for in their own right.

Psychotherapy may be given individually, that is, with just the patient and therapist present, or it may be given simultaneously to a group of patients. Individual psychotherapy may sometimes help to overcome the diffidence of patients whose self-esteem at the outset is especially low. It may concentrate on giving them an understanding of the psychological reasons for their being unable to cope with certain recurrent situations in life. It can help them to understand their anxieties, to appreciate how unhelpful is their recourse to alcohol and to develop new psychological strengths to dispel or overcome them. Frequently they gain insight into their personal psychological make-up in the process.

Sessions can last from fifteen to fifty minutes and can take place weekly or more often. The atmosphere during each interview should be as supportive as possible; the patient will often suffer great distress when speaking of harrowing experiences. Actual details of setting, timing and frequency have to depend, of course, on the individual circumstances of the patient, and to some extent on the availability of the therapist's time and the type of psychotherapy he or she chooses to follow.

Group therapy

Group therapy is widely advocated in the treatment of alcoholics, because it has been found both more acceptable to patients and equally effective.

The members of a treatment group, generally about six to ten alcoholics, meet with one psychiatrist for sessions of an hour and a half each week, for about a year. The psychiatrist who has chosen patients whom he or she considers suitable to form a particular group conducts the meetings so as to evoke group interactions which bring about personality changes.

A group session consists of the descriptions by members of their recent experiences, each one speaking as they wish, when they consider they have an idea to contribute to the discussion.

As the weeks pass, the members of the group report and pool their experiences; small triumphs are noted and disasters are shared, not only with interested attention but with responsible concern, because any member's set-back is thoroughly understood and may perhaps even have been anticipated. When a member has a lapse and begins to drink, the skills developed by the group are put to the test; understanding, firmness in reaching sound decisions and skill in communicating them often help the drinking member to recover sobriety without incurring serious harm.

Alcoholics in a group are able to try out new ways of approaching people, secure in the knowledge that the reactions of fellow members, whether appreciative or critical, will never be scornful or humiliating. Because of their personal experience of the illness they can say things about each other that they would not so well tolerate hearing from non-alcoholics. Moreover, they know that the therapist conducting the group will control the development of individual or group emotions too threatening or too disruptive for the members themselves to handle. The therapist trained in group methods conducts the meetings so as to foster therapeutic interactions and to ensure that harmful developments are recognized in time and promptly checked and counteracted. The role does not call for domination of the group or for giving advice. The group collectively works through the conflicts of opinion between members, and other problems which arise as private preoccupations are disclosed and discussed.

As they gain in self-confidence, unassertive alcoholics discover that to express themselves forcefully does not incur the catastrophes they had previously feared. In this way patients learn to understand the motives for their behaviour and develop ways of modifying them when they are unrealistic, and their chances of subsequently remaining abstinent even when difficulties arise are greatly strengthened.

A former accountant in a group found employment as time-keeper on a building site. He had taken care to let his employers know of his alcoholism. His foreman told him to mark as present a man whom he was illicitly sending elsewhere. This happened repeatedly. The patient discussed his difficulty in his treatment group. As he saw it, he would have to refuse but he was certain the foreman would see to it that he lost his hard-found job. The group members sympathetically agreed that here was a perplexing problem; although individual members offered differing advice the consensus was that he should do what the foreman instructed. He did the opposite. His rebellion against the group's opinion was a try-out for subsequent rebellion against the foreman. He told the foreman that he was not happy about marking the absentee present. 'You do as I tell you,' said the foreman threateningly. Very unhappily he obeyed, but his protest was successful. The foreman never again asked him to be dishonest. This achievement gave him the confidence he needed to tell his employers that he was really capable of a more exacting job.

During the course of a group session, problems will be focused upon, generally arising out of a recent situation related by one member, who also tells how he or she reacted to it. This becomes a theme in the discussion and it is worked upon from all sides. A patient described a lapse into drinking: 'I fell away last week. I'm having trouble with my daughter. I'd finished my Antabuse and intended to get more at last week's meeting.' His wife, he said, had urged him to take their daughter to task. At first she had supported him when he began to reprimand the girl but then, 'as she usually does when she thinks I become too harsh with the children, my wife changed over and sided with my daughter. I couldn't stand that. I went out, had a couple of whiskies, and then came home to continue the brawl.'

Mr Peel said that he also had difficulty with his children because he was not sure how to deal with them.

'You can't dictate to young people today,' said Mr Fox. 'They think for themselves. You can't tie them down, especially the girls.'

Mr Walpole, the original speaker, could not accept this: 'I'm not going to stand for it. If she comes back home late again she'll find the door shut.' 'What right have we to judge our children?' asked Mr Fox, and the group went on to consider, some of them for the first time, how their children might understandably be confused by not knowing what value to place upon admonitions and controls exercised by a parent who until recently had been disorganized by drinking.

Mr Walpole admitted reflectively that his daughter had indeed been concerned about him when he was drinking. 'But,' he went on, 'a father *has* to exercise control. Once you let the children get on top of you, that's it.'

The group continued to discuss the position of the alcoholic parent. 'When you were drinking it didn't matter what time your daughter came in. The child thinks: "He didn't care before, why should he care now?" ' They insisted to Mr Walpole that aggressive handling of his daughter would fail. 'If you come the heavy father, she'll just go off.' Another member, Mrs Holland, introduced a new note when she talked about her own youth. 'At sixteen I used to stay out late.' She said that, like Mr Walpole's wife, 'I want my husband to chastise the children if they do wrong, but when he does I take their side against him.' Several of the men then said that their wives also placed them in this false position. Mrs Holland, by identifying herself with Mr Walpole's wife, had taken on the role of all the missing spouses. But she was herself an alcoholic, so she could express the group's problem, which she did precisely: 'I tell my boy to be in by ten o'clock or there will be a row, and he answers back, "You weren't in by ten when you were in the pubs." Then there is chaos.'

Each member of the group had become enabled to see how his or her own actions in a common situation appeared to others, to spouses and to children. Relationships, in particular between parents and children, were no longer seen as one-sided. Now they were putting themselves imaginatively in the position of their children, trying to see themselves from the outside. This led Mr Peel, whose father was also an alcoholic, to conclude with feeling: 'I mean to be different to my children than my father was to me.' The group had done its work for that session but the therapist had registered a possible clue to Mr Walpole's intractable harshness to his daughter; he decided that he would provide an opportunity in a later session for Mr Walpole to discuss the treatment he had received from his father, which might be serving as a model for his own behaviour as a parent.

The group process does three things. It supports recovering alcoholics in their abstinence by letting them see that they are wrong to think that being an alcoholic is sinful and degenerate. When they perceive the strengths and positive capacities of their fellow patients, disgust with themselves also diminishes. When they see that others accomplish what they feared was impossible they begin to believe that they can themselves reorganize their lives to exclude alcohol. Secondly it shows them the situations in which they repeatedly involve themselves but which they characteristically mismanage, so that they learn to deal with them more effectively. Lastly, group members, by examining their and other members' ways of reacting, and by exploring the origins of those ways, can in time modify their self-defeating patterns of behaviour.

Follow-up

No treatment regime is complete that does not involve following patients up to make sure that they are progressing well and to intervene swiftly if relapse into drinking occurs. Alcoholism is a relapsing condition. Both the therapeutic team and the alcoholics themselves and their families have to accept this. All too often, those who relapse are made to feel (in this they will need little encouragement) that they have failed and, what is worse, failed their helpers. As a result they may be too ashamed to seek help from them again. It has to be impressed on each patient being treated both that recommencement of drinking need not constitute total disaster, and that it is the conjunction of patient and treater that has jointly not yet done well enough.

The Team Approach

We have now covered the three areas of a treatment programme; dealing with the alcohol itself, coping with life problems and strengthening the psychological abilities of the alcoholic. This puts us in a good position to consider how a team functions to treat alcoholics. The principal professions involved are doctor, social worker, nurse and clinical psychologist. It is uncommon for all four to be needed in the treatment of any one patient, but they may all have to put their heads together to decide who should play the leading part.

The Clinical Psychologist

Clinical psychologists (who are not medically qualified) may be asked to assess the degree of any psychological deficits that have been wrought by alcohol upon a patient's brain. Thus they may have to assess the current level of intellectual functioning of the patient and, in particular, determine whether there has been any significant memory loss. This they do by carrying out specific tests, which cannot be properly performed until the patient is free from the immediate effects of alcohol in the body and is not undergoing any withdrawal symptoms.

Some clinical psychologists consider that the whole of alcohol dependence can be viewed as merely a learned bad habit. They aim to treat the condition, therefore, merely by habit-breaking techniques. This method of treatment virtually ignores the alcoholic and his or her problems and concentrates on habit-breaking. Excessive drinking is what they deal with rather than alcoholism. Indeed they do not care to employ that term. They see excessive drinking as a piece of learned behaviour that is not serving the individual well, and they use a variety of conditioning techniques to break the habit. This reductionist view of alcoholism does not do justice to the number of factors involved in causing alcoholism and might not, therefore, in itself be a sufficient form of treatment.

The Nurse

Nurse responsibility in treating alcoholics is growing. Naturally, if the patient is admitted to hospital specially for the treatment of alcoholism, nurses are inevitably involved and may well play a part in the psychotherapy, whether individual or group, as well as with day-to-day routine care. Recently, *community psychiatric nurses* have been appointed in increasing numbers. Such nurses, especially as less and less of treatment occurs inside hospitals, have come to play an ever growing role both in following up and supporting patients but also in carrying out psychotherapy to the full extent that their training makes possible. The nurses' ready availability without the patient having to report to hospital gives an added advantage to their therapeutic role.

The Social Worker

Social workers can play the major role in the treatment of some alcoholics, especially if their training has equipped them with the necessary combination of skills both to help sort out the patients' predicaments with their environment and to provide individual therapy. Apart from their skills, social workers sometimes have the advantage of seeming less an authority figure than the doctor does.

The Doctor

The doctor involved may be the *general practitioner* (of whose particular role more later); a gastroenterologist, when the patient arrives at hospital with symptoms of illness in the stomach or digestive tract; an accident and emergency doctor, when the patient comes to the casualty department of the hospital either suffering from collapse from intoxication or following a drunken accident; or indeed a specialist in any other branch of medicine. These specialists are called on to do three things only: to recognize that the cause is alcoholism (unfortunately there is abundant evidence that they frequently fail to do this), to persuade the patient that he or she needs treatment, and to refer them for such treatment to their general practitioner or to a psychiatrist.

The Psychiatrist

Psychiatrists are the specialist doctors principally concerned in treatment, and they will have received special training to that end. They are equipped to recognize all the medical aspects of alcoholism, although they may consult with specialists about particular decisions, and they will be able to supervise the period of alcohol withdrawal, initiate treatment with Antabuse or Abstem and initiate and carry out psychotherapy. More importantly, they will be able to set up any necessary investigations and devise, with the patient, the treatment plan. They should be able to call on the resources of a treatment team as described above and to seek their advice and help. However, the large number of alcoholics compared to the small number of psychiatrists means, in practice, that the psychiatrist will, in many instances, be offering an investigation and assessment of the situation to the referring general practitioner together with advice to this family doctor about treatment that the latter will be carrying out. Of course he or she will make plain a willingness to see the patient again whenever necessary. Because of their clinical role, psychiatrists may be the people who initially explain matters not only to patients but also to husbands and wives. They may also be called upon to write letters on the patient's behalf to the courts, to housing authorities and sometimes to the police. One of the essential roles for psychiatrists is to be seen by the alcoholic to be taking charge of the situation. It is important that they adopt an expectant attitude, that is, that they appear always to be expressing confidence in the patient's capacity to improve. They may not scruple to tell the patient, as bluntly as necessary, what may happen if he or she continues to drink. They can be, and should sound, optimistic about what the outcome would be if the patient were to cease to drink and accept the other necessary treatment. This is not false optimism. Improvement is rightly to be expected, even though cure of damage already done may be less possible.

The Expert in Alcoholism

Some psychiatrists have had extra training specifically in the field of alcoholism to prepare them for the planning and management of special alcoholism services. In Britain there are only between thirty and fifty such psychiatrists, and they are often to be found in charge of alcoholism treatment units, which we shall shortly describe. Such psychiatrists spend much of their time developing a network of services to recognize, treat and care for alcoholics. They are available to advise other psychiatrists and to take over the treatment of particularly complicated and difficult patients. They form the third medical tier: general practitioner, psychiatrist, special expert: but they cannot themselves treat more than a tiny minority of patients.

How the Team Work Together

The team of doctor, nurse, social worker and psychologist work together inasmuch as they meet as a team and devise and implement the strategy of treatment to suit the alcoholic's particular needs: whether, for instance, to concentrate most on social work or on psychotherapy – thus deciding which member should be seeing the patient in an ongoing relationship. As the team members soon come to understand what each of the others is able to contribute they may not all need to consider each alcoholic who comes to one or other of them; nevertheless, whoever first sees the alcoholic will refer to his or her colleagues for any relevant help. They know they have each other's backing, just as the general practitioners know that they can call on members of the team to support their treatment.

We turn now to some special issues concerning treatment, and to some special methods or services that may play a part in the overall treatment of an alcoholic.

Where the Alcoholic Should be Treated

The first issue concerns whether a patient needs to be admitted to hospital in order to have treatment. Sometimes, as we have noted, the objective of treatment is simply to secure such an admission so that the alcoholic is safely housed and does not endanger his or her life. Sometimes admission is needed because of physical illness or because withdrawal symptoms become severe. Alternatively it can become necessary because the patient is depressed and there is suicidal risk, or perhaps there is such severe brain damage or psychosis that admission is required on that ground. Sometimes the patients are living on their own and need the head start to treatment that being away from temptation provides. Yet in the majority of instances, where the alcoholic is not physically damaged and retains a reasonable social hold, experts in alcoholism are finding that admission to hospital provides few advantages and, indeed, some disadvantages, chief of which is that the thought of admission is a disincentive to accepting treatment. Nowadays we find that the matter is best dealt with by discussion with the patients themselves. If they want to enter hospital, then a place is offered. If they do not, we tend to see how it goes on an out-patient basis. We can always review the situation if excessive drinking continues. Sometimes a patient can be asked to attend as a day patient, that is, to attend for some time during each day from Monday to Friday, or perhaps two or three times in the week. This permits full assessment of the history and current status of the patient. Unfortunately, it does not cover evening opening hours of drinking establishments; nevertheless it works well for some patients.

Recently it has been shown that one single day's attendance as an out-patient, during which assessment is carried out in a concentrated way, and advice offered, achieves as good a result as admitting the patient for a long period. This is discussed in the next chapter. As a general rule we do not often admit patients today who still have a home and family and who are not physically damaged. Certainly the days are over when it was thought ideal to admit patients for up to three months in order to build up their physical and psychological strength and social stability. Patients are rarely asked to stay for more than three weeks, including the period of detoxification.

Compulsory Detention

Some people argue (they are rarely experts in the matter) that as alcoholics endanger their health and indeed their lives, it is reasonable to use the compulsory powers that exist under the Mental Health Act to make patients enter hospital and compel them to stay there. We do not in any way support that view. First, we very much doubt whether it is possible to stretch the Mental Health Act to permit this. Secondly, it is useless to attempt to treat patients for alcoholism compulsorily, against their will. Indeed it may be worse than useless, for it will forfeit the patient's cooperation, probably for all time. Nor would it be proper. If, as a result of alcoholism, or coincident with it, the alcoholic has a mental illness which in its own right justifies the use of compulsory detention powers, then that is another matter, but they should not be used merely to deal with the alcoholism.

Decriminalizing Alcoholism

In the last ten or fifteen years there has been a lot of discussion about whether alcoholism should be *decriminalized*, that is to say, making public drunkenness of a minor nature, such as being drunk and disorderly, no longer an offence and hence no longer a matter for the police. We do not consider that any useful purpose is served by submitting drunken people to the legal process, but at least the police do pick them up from the street and provide shelter for them, albeit overnight in the cells. They see to it that they do not lie in, or drown in, their own vomit, and that medical help is sought when it is seen to be required. If such attention to drunken people is to be taken out of police hands, it is imperative that, before changes are made in the law to that effect, some other provision is made for their care. Otherwise they will die in the streets. Casualty departments of hospitals are ill-equipped to handle instances of alcohol intoxication and are under-resourced for them. Staff in these busy departments are unhappy at receiving such patients and, consequently, often unfriendly if not actively hostile. One cannot blame them. Having to deal with an uncooperative and perhaps obstreperous drunken patient whilst sick and injured people are also needing attention is hardly likely to foster a caring attitude to the alcoholic.

Detoxification Centres

Recently, in response to government initiatives in Britain, some experimental detoxification centres were set up. They had three principal purposes: first, to prevent alcoholics, apprehended simply for public drunkenness, from having to go through the degrading and therapeutically useless rigmarole of appearance in court; second, to cover alcoholic withdrawal and assess the long-term treatment needs of each patient; and third, to induce them to enter a treatment programme once the acute situation had been dealt with. One of us was closely concerned with a detoxification centre in a general hospital and associated with an alcohol treatment unit. Research evaluation[34] showed that the majority of alcoholics picked up by the police could not be brought to the centre, or did not wish to come or, when they came, did not stay. Those who stayed and were assessed developed much less in the way of withdrawal symptoms than predicted. We believe this was because police referrals contained a higher proportion of intermittent rather than regular heavy drinkers than had been anticipated; there were more withdrawal symptoms among intoxicated patients sent by general practitioners, but even these patients did not usually need medication. Our patients also showed very little in the way of physical illnesses requiring urgent intervention or of abnormal mental states. Chronic illness, when it was present, was rarely serious enough to warrant in-patient treatment. Finally, relatively few patients agreed to go on to anti-alcoholism treatment. If they did agree, they did not actually arrive at it, or, if they went, they did not stay. From a detailed follow-up study we were forced to conclude that those few patients who showed any long-term benefit following their admission to the detoxification unit did so because of the support given as part of the follow-up procedure rather than because of treatment received. While it may prevent a misuse of police cells and hospital emergency departments and thus be administratively tidy to channel intoxicated patients to a detoxification service, such a service certainly does not need to be in a hospital, where it is inevitably expensive to run. Also, there is no evidence that going to such a centre has any effect upon the long-term outcome. Shelters in city centres, run by voluntary agencies but with medical help rapidly available, are what is needed.

Alcoholism Treatment Units

Alcoholism Treatment Units were set up in Britain from the 1950s onwards, and there is now one in most large towns. They are highly specialized units where all the four professional disciplines concerned with treatment work together. Their purpose is not to provide treatment for all alcoholics in their vicinity. They do, of course, treat a lot of alcoholics, but their main function is to develop services of all sorts within the community for the treatment of alcoholism and to treat patients who present particular difficulties. They also have an important educational role. Recently much of their work has moved from in-patient care to out-patient work and the development of links with community services.

Hostels

A network of hostels now exists in Britain – far too few, of course, to cope with the need. Sometimes these are run by statutory, but more usually by voluntary, agencies. They range in purpose from therapeutic units that carry out all anti-alcoholism treatment plans that do not require medical services, to shelters for the care of derelict and physically decrepit individuals. Some are dry hostels, where drinking on the premises, or returning to them in a drunken state, is not permitted and leads to the patient being discharged. These dry hostels often act as the next stage of the treatment of alcoholics who have been detoxified or otherwise treated in hospital. Some are wet hostels, which receive alcoholics for whom sobriety is an impossible aim. Some expect patients to pass fairly rapidly through them to go on to live independent lives; others know that the alcoholics who come there are likely to stay, if not for ever, at least for a considerable time. Almost all hostels aim to provide an element of stability in the alcoholics' otherwise storm-tossed lives.

Alcoholics Anonymous

The inspired plan to help alcoholics by enabling them to help other alcoholics was devised by a stockbroker, Bill W., and a medical practitioner, Dr Bob, at Akron, Ohio, in 1935. The movement was based on concepts and techniques derived from a number of sources. Both founders were active Oxford Group members and used as a basis for Alcoholics Anonymous the principles of open self-scrutiny, admission of defects, aid to others, and making reparations for harm done in the past. The religious component is epitomized by their adoption of an eighteenth-century prayer of Friedrich Ötinger: 'God give me the detachment to accept those things I cannot alter; the courage to alter those things which I can alter; and the wisdom to distinguish the ones from the others'; AA members, in a phrase of William James, are asked in Step Two to believe that 'a Power greater than ourselves' can restore them to sanity. The physician W. D. Silkworth proposed to the founders of the movement the idea that alcoholism was an illness; his belief that the basis of the condition was an allergy to alcohol was enthusiastically adopted and widely publicized.[35] Bill Wilson wrote to the psychoanalyst Carl Jung in June 1961[36] about Silkworth:

> It was his theory that alcoholism had two components – an obsession that compelled the sufferer to drink against his will and interest, and some sort of metabolism difficulty which he then called an allergy. The alcoholic's compulsion guaranteed that the alcoholic's drinking

would go on, and the 'allergy' made sure that the sufferer would finally deteriorate, go insane, or die.

This, as we have seen, is no longer a tenable hypothesis, but it permitted an approach to be formulated which identifies the drinking itself as the disease process. Stopping drinking and remaining abstinent are the goals of AA members. In their theoretical statement of the causes of alcoholism they do not adopt the broader approach of the medical profession, which holds that there are underlying psychological factors to which attention must be paid.

Their programme is based on the famous Twelve Steps:

We –

1. Admitted we were powerless over alcohol – that our lives had become unmanageable.

2. Came to believe that a Power greater than ourselves could restore us to sanity.

3. Made a decision to turn our will and our lives over to the care of God as we understood Him.

4. Made a searching and fearless moral inventory of ourselves.

5. Admitted to God, to ourselves, and to another human being, the exact nature of our wrongs.

6. Were entirely ready to have God remove all these defects of character.

7. Humbly asked Him to remove our shortcomings.

8. Made a list of all persons we had harmed and became willing to make amends to them all.

9. Made direct amends to such people wherever possible, except when to do so would injure them or others.

10. Continued to take a personal inventory and when we were wrong promptly admitted it.

11. Sought through power of prayer and meditation to improve our conscious contact with God as we understood Him, praying only for knowledge of His will for us and the power to carry that out.

12. Having had a spiritual experience as a result of these steps, tried to carry this message to alcoholics and to practise these principles in all our affairs.

These steps are buttressed by twelve 'Traditions', which are concerned with the cohesion and management of local groups. The first tradition is: 'Our common welfare should come first; personal recovery depends on AA unity.' The fifth tradition runs: 'Each group has but one primary purpose – to carry its message to the alcoholic who still suffers.' The ninth takes us firmly into the organizational sphere: 'Alcoholics Anonymous has no opinion on outside issues; hence the AA name ought never be drawn into public controversy.'

To join, all one has to do is get in touch with any AA member or look them up in the telephone directory; there are groups in most cities. Anybody who wants to stop drinking and is prepared to admit that they are 'powerless over alcohol' can join AA. Alcoholics who join a group are provided with a new subculture, made up of companions engaged upon a common task.[37] Only alcoholics play a part in the movement, which does not rely on doctors or ministers or other professional personnel (unless they are themselves alcoholics). A new, all-embracing outlook on life is offered them. They learn a special, memorable, technical language in which to talk about and reflect on the symptoms occurring in the course of alcoholism, and they absorb a system of ideas devised by alcoholics themselves to provide practical ways of becoming abstinent. 'Sobriety date' is the time at which an AA member last had a drink. An 'oldtimer' is an AA regular with ten years or more continuous sobriety. 'Serenity' is an AA term for peace of mind, emotional equanimity and the absence of negativity in one's life. At the meetings members describe their successes and failures since the last meeting and discuss difficulties common to all. A new member may be introduced and absent members may be inquired about. One or more members will usually relate the story of former drinking days and successful recovery.

As the designation of Alcoholics Anonymous emphasizes, anonymity is strictly preserved. First names only are used, so that members can shed some of the customary social caution. (In English AA groups more stress than in North America is placed on the anonymity principle.)[38]

Each newcomer is assigned a sponsor, an AA member who has

successfully stopped drinking. The function of the sponsor is to come to the sufferer's aid whenever necessary and to stay with them for as long as necessary. The care and selflessness shown by some sponsors is one of the twin pillars of the movement, the other being the group meetings, which may occur as often as every night.

The success of different AA groups in providing active sponsorship for new members and in dealing with rivalries, open hostilities and other quarrelsome behaviour varies from group to group.[39]

Alcoholics who succeed with AA's help in becoming abstinent have found a constant body of people who share their enduring interest to stay sober regardless of difficulties which crop up. The discovery of so many pleasant men and women in the group helps them considerably in ridding themselves of the idea that alcoholics, themselves in particular, are despicable. Their own self-esteem grows with this realization. They find friends, an active social life, the satisfaction of helping others and, in time, the chance to take a leading part in the affairs of their local group. Their guilt over the harm they did to others is reduced both by the relief of confession and by the opportunities for reparation which they are afforded when called upon to sponsor new members. Many AA members find that the movement becomes their overriding life concern.

The AA approach can be a life-changing experience for alcoholics who are sociable, who derive satisfaction from helping fellow sufferers and from their company, who are responsive to concentrated attention upon drinking and who do not seek psychological exploration and treatment of underlying problems.

Nowadays AA has come to work closely with most other agencies that treat alcoholics, and in most alcoholism treatment units members of AA come to visit, are introduced to patients who are interested, and may even conduct meetings. AA is now regarded as a partner in treatment, not a rival. Equally AA has come to accept that medical and other services may have a valuable role that it cannot itself perform.

AA achieves least success with those alcoholics who are not

gregarious and cannot tolerate the pressures towards continuous and intimate relationships with others. Such alcoholics mention this as one of their chief reasons for not having been helped by the movement. Another is the distaste that may be engendered not only by having to confess publicly about their drinking history but also by the apparent relish with which, one after another, hardened abstainers recount their past and rehearse their former drinking habits.

These activities together with the religious emphasis, which varies considerably from group to group, put off some newcomers who feel themselves not part of the group. They are undoubtedly features which may strike an outsider attending an open meeting as unacceptable; however, the movement is not intended for outsiders but for insiders. It has forged techniques which it has found effective for many alcoholics. AA realizes, for instance, that public declarations of former drinking act as a necessary group defence against relapse, by serving as a constant reminder of what might happen again.

Recently other voluntary agencies have entered the field of helping alcoholics – Accept is a good example – by offering services and support from helpers who are not necessarily ex-alcoholics.

Two forms of treatment for alcoholism that are still sometimes discussed but which are hardly ever used now, and which we certainly do not use in our own work, merit a brief account.

Aversion Treatment

Alcoholism can be treated by a method of *conditioning*. The essential of such a procedure is to induce in the patient an extremely unpleasant sensation in response to the taste, smell, and sight of alcohol. We will describe the most commonly used method, employing the drug apomorphine. This has only one important medical property: when injected it acts on the brain centres to produce vomiting.

Treatment consists of giving the patient alcohol in conjunction with an injection, carefully timed so that nausea begins very shortly after the drink is taken and the patient vomits. The procedure is repeated several times in the course of a treatment session and half a dozen sessions take place over the course of about a fortnight. By the end of the conditioning course the patient has built up nauseating associations to the smell, taste, and gastric effects of alcohol. The conditioning stimulus of apomorphine is no longer necessary. The patient develops nausea whenever a drink is handled. In order to reinforce the conditioning, further treatment courses are advised, initially at six-monthly intervals but less frequently later on.

The treatment is drastic. It can only be administered under strict medical supervision since it is necessary that means should be available for combating collapse in those few patients who may be prostrated by the vomiting. Emetine is another drug sometimes used to induce vomiting.

More recently other agents have been used to produce a conditioned response. Patients have been induced to associate the effects of drinking with the pain of electric shocks or with sudden muscle paralysis which follows the injection of muscle-relaxants of the curare type.

Clinicians in Britain and in North America have not been drawn to the use of methods which involve submitting their patients to unpleasant and painful procedures. There are other forms of medical treatment, surgery for instance, in which the patient is necessarily hurt, but the doctor tries to minimize the pain as much as possible. In aversion treatment the suffering of the patient is deliberately brought about by the doctor. Alcoholics who submit to this treatment must be prodigiously well motivated to overcome their addiction. In Britain it is chiefly practised outside the National Health Service. The chief exponent of aversion therapy in the United States, who uses apomorphine, claims recovery for half his patients, who come mostly from the upper social classes and were able to pay for private treatment.[40]

There is no doubt that aversion therapy is quick, that it is safe under controlled conditions, and that it is based on a consistent psychological theory resting on firm experimental evidence. On the other hand, many physicians will continue to find it unacceptable and it ignores all the psychological factors determining alcoholism.

Hypnosis

Alcoholics sometimes ask to be treated by hypnosis, and this has been employed by a few physicians. The basis of the method is to suggest to alcoholics either that they do not enjoy drinking or else that drink makes them sick. Such suggestions, however, do not prove to be lasting, and few, if any, alcoholics have been permanently helped by treatment which depends principally on this approach.

The Proper Course of Action

Now that we have reviewed the types of treatment that are, or should be, available, we can see how alcoholics may take stock of their position once they have realized that they are alcoholics and that they need help to recover. What steps can they take? They can contact the local branch of AA or go to their doctor and state the problem bluntly. Nor should they be satisfied until they are receiving expert care. They should expect a general hospital to undertake all the treatment of their physical complications and to accept them as patients during the process of detoxification when they first stop drinking and withdrawal symptoms occur. They should expect the psychiatrist who becomes responsible for any subsequent hospital management to design a programme to suit the requirements of the case. This should offer a positive approach to alcoholism during the period of in-patient care, in which the skills of the psychiatrist, psychiatric social worker and nursing staff are each deployed. It is of the greatest importance that every alcoholic should be enabled to learn the facts about alcoholism as an illness. This is one of our purposes in writing this book.

During the subsequent out-patient treatment the same personnel will consolidate the treatment gains. They will help the patients further to achieve the personal integration that will enable them to lead their lives profitably without further recourse to alcohol. If they should suffer a relapse they are entitled to expect that the staff concerned will not give them up but will rally to their support with a renewed offer of their resources.

If they do not find all this, they are not getting the treatment they deserve and that the illness deserves.

Chapter 11

Results of Treatment

What are the chances of an alcoholic stopping drinking? What are the benefits of treatment? Since the objectives of treatment differ for different groups of alcoholics there can be no universal criterion of success. Further, alcoholic patients can be very difficult to follow up because many of them, especially those in advanced stages, have no fixed abode and move around a lot; tracing them becomes virtually impossible. If reports of a follow-up study are based only upon those actually followed up, the results will seem much rosier than if all patients treated were included, although it is wrong to go to the other extreme and assume that all those not traced were treatment failures. Lastly, if one is assessing the successes or failures of treatment, there really should be a comparison group of people who were not treated. For ethical and other reasons this is next to impossible to obtain.

We have seen that involuntary abstinence is fairly simply achieved by placing the drinker in hospital or prison. There are no studies to tell us whether any of these people remain abstinent afterwards, but experience suggests that there must be very few such cases indeed. Temporary compulsory removal from sources of supply is not by itself an effective treatment for alcohol addiction.

Many alcoholics stop drinking with the help of Alcoholics Anonymous, but its very anonymity militates against the production of checkable statistics of recovery.

We can, however, obtain some information from reports of the success or failure of certain treatment programmes. Abstinence is the customary yardstick of success that is used in investigations following up treated alcoholics. However, it is wrong to view abstinence as the only index of recovery or improvement: that is too limited a perspective. Some abstinent alcoholics are still disturbed people, as we will discuss later on, though previous claims that a number of treated alcoholics can continue to drink socially and improve their adjustment in other respects are now discredited.[41] However, as in the case of chronic alcoholics with advanced physical disease and social disorganization, the correct objective of treatment may only be to improve as far as possible their physical conditions and to provide them with shelter.

A number of early investigations set out to determine whether or not treated alcoholics resumed drinking. Many follow-up studies, carried out with varying degrees of rigour, have been made. The advantage of abstinence as a criterion has been that it is an absolute measure, whereas the extent of drinking is not. Research workers have also considered social adjustment, and, to a lesser extent, general well-being.

Planned Care

When planned treatment is provided, the outcome is better. Davies and his colleagues[42] studied fifty cases at the Maudsley Hospital in London, where treatment of alcoholics was provided in a ward admitting all types of psychiatric patient. The treatment plan was geared to the individual patient's requirements; Antabuse, social work and individual psychotherapy were the treatment methods, following out-patient treatment on a supportive basis. Two years later, 18 per cent were found to be totally abstinent and another 18 per cent had been abstinent for most of the time, while 42 per cent of the patients had maintained their social efficiency despite light or heavy drinking. The outcome at six months accurately predicted the two-year outcome.

Glatt[43] reported on 150 alcoholics treated as voluntary patients at Warlingham Park Hospital, near London. A third became totally abstinent. Another third relapsed, usually within six months, but were rated as improved because they were drinking less and in better social circumstances. A third of the patients were treatment failures.

Costello[44] has reviewed fifty-eight investigations reporting a follow-up at least one year after treatment. These studies covered 11,022 treated alcoholics, using outcome measures that were not confined just to abstinence but also credited controlled drinking or drinking without recurrence of problems. The overall conclusions that he drew from these studies were that about a quarter were classified as improved, a half were still drinking with associated problems after a one-year post-treatment period, and a fifth could not be traced. One per cent were dead. Costello[45] also reviewed twenty-three investigations into the outcome of treatment of alcoholism followed up for two years, comprising 5,833 alcoholics: 35 per cent were found definitely improved, 43 per cent were still drinking with problems, 19 per cent could not be traced, and 3 per cent were dead. These studies reported by Costello were for all forms of treatment.

Again, the overall remission rate six months after the initiation of treatment predicted quite accurately the rate of remission at later periods of follow-up.

Emrick looked only at treatments that, for the most part, relied on a psychiatric or psychological approach. Pooling such studies together,[46] he found that half the patients had achieved total abstinence, and two thirds were rated as having demonstrated some improvement. Of course we can expect that patients selected for psychological treatments were likely not to have been so far down the road to chronic alcoholism as unselected patients.

There are pointers to the types of patients most likely to succeed in treatment. Earlier studies reported that women fared worse than men; however, we are far from sure that this is the case today. Older men, so long as they are not physically deteriorated, do better than younger men. Social stability, especially having a job, is associated with a better outcome from treatment. Married people do better than those who are single or divorced. Patients with psychopathic personality disorder, that is, anti-social people, who experience little subjective distress themselves but cause others to suffer, respond poorly to treatment. Patients who seem to the treatment staff to be lacking in cooperation, who surreptitiously drink while in hospital, and who do not respond constructively to psychological explorations, are more likely to relapse into drinking after treatment. Those who are well motivated for treatment are much more likely to become abstinent.

Not every patient conforms to these statistical generalizations. Some patients who are not cooperative, who resist efforts of the treatment staff to help them, and who make no substantial modification in their pattern of living, sometimes confound prediction by remaining abstinent.

There have been a few studies which attempted to analyse the outcome in minimally treated or untreated alcoholics. There is without doubt a spontaneous remission rate which is not negligible. Patients who were given no more than custodial care in a mental hospital were followed up six years later; of ninety-eight who had been committed to Michigan State Hospital, eighteen were found to have become abstinent and a further sixteen were drinking only 'moderately'.[47] When Emrick[48] looked at seven studies in which alcoholics received no treatment at all he found that half were improved, and 13 per cent of these were abstinent. In seventeen studies of really minimal treatment, 21 per cent became abstinent and over 60 per cent (the abstinent included) were somewhat improved. In all these studies the follow-up was of at least six months' duration. These studies may be reporting different types of patients, but they certainly show that considerable improvement can occur without treatment. That recovery can be independent of treatment has been shown in other large studies.

Is Return to Social Drinking Possible?

Whenever treatment goals are discussed, patients sooner or later ask whether they must aim at abstinence or whether they might be able to resume drinking at some reduced level within social norms. It used to be held by all experts that alcoholics had to give up drinking completely; if after attaining abstinence they began drinking again they would inexorably relapse into their former excessive drinking habits. Then in 1962 Davies[49] reported that seven out of ninety-three patients had, after ceasing treatment, begun social drinking again without escalating the amount. This is the secret hope of all alcoholics. Davies's work attracted much comment. Alcoholic experts mostly condemned it: it was not news that they wanted to hear or that they wished their patients to hear. Davies also reported that he had not been able to predict, either from the histories of his patients or from how they had behaved under treatment, which patients could safely begin drinking and which could not. We should add that almost all patients believe that they are one of the group that can learn to drink socially. Davies's findings have been replicated in other investigations. Armor et al.,[50] in a review of some of the patients from forty-four alcoholism treatment centres in the United States, found that 12 per cent seemed to be drinking normally – that is, with an average daily consumption of less than three ounces of alcohol, and no tremor or serious symptoms. Such quantities, however, still would place people in a high risk group for future trouble. An interesting succession of reports began with Sobell and Sobell[51] claiming that they had succeeded in 'shaping' alcoholics in their experiment to practise controlled social drinking after treatment. Caddy et al.[52] re-studied this same group of alcoholics in an additional follow-up three years after treatment and confirmed the Sobells' claims. But Pendery et al.[53] revealingly re-examined the alcoholics reported in the Sobells' study and discovered that thirteen of the first sixteen subjects had been rehospitalized for alcoholism treatment approximately one year after discharge. The long-term drinking histories of the twenty subjects, over ten years up to 1981, showed that one alcoholic who had controlled his drinking after the end of the first year was still doing so; eight were drinking excessively and regularly; six were abstaining but only after multiple hospitalizations for alcoholism; and four of the controlled drinking subjects eventually died alcohol-related deaths.

Almost all those who begin drinking again soon revert to excessive drinking. Some patients with alcoholism return to normal social drinking. However, since it is impossible to predict who will manage it, the advice must be to aim for abstinence.

Outcome of Different Types of Treatment

There is need for considerable experiment with different treatment methods. Many studies confirm what we have stated, namely that well-motivated patients do better than poorly motivated ones. Social work involvement is associated with a good outcome; so is out-patient follow-up. In addition, behaviour therapy and the use of Antabuse go with a good outcome. Poor results are associated with taking unselected patients into treatment, meagre treatment resources and treating large numbers of patients.[54]

Patients who received little treatment have been compared in terms of outcome with those who went through extended programmes. An important study by Orford and Edwards[55] reported that one day's exceptionally intensive out-patient assessment and advice yielded as good results as admission to an alcoholism treatment unit programme.

Chick and his colleagues at Edinburgh[56] randomly assigned alcoholics either to one session of advice or to extended inpatient or outpatient treatment. Two years later the group who had extended treatment were functioning better, accumulating less harm to themselves, their families and society than those only treated briefly. Abstinence was not, however, more common in patients given extended treatment.

The more research there is in the area of treatment the better. At the moment many agencies with differing professional backgrounds and different orientations towards the care of the alcoholic practise treatment without assessing their treatment results. Sometimes this may be unavoidable, as with Alcoholics Anonymous, but it is often inexcusable: some treatment services seem quite prepared to practise their methods apparently without ever recognizing the need to question whether they are effective. In other places assessments are made with such a lack of scientific rigour that their purported successes are unconvincing. Many agencies carry out no follow-up of their treated cases. How can they know whether the alcoholics remained abstinent, or continued to drink but improved physically and socially? With scarcely more sophistication, others have observed the remission rate as a percentage of those who responded to an inquiry, ignoring those who had escaped their follow-up and who might very well have relapsed. It can be very misleading to take an alcoholic's statements of sobriety at face value, without seeking corroboration. There are many agencies which depend for their admirable work on public funds and issue optimistic and nebulous reports of their successes, often providing an illustrative case history or two. They do a disservice by underplaying the difficulties in providing adequate treatment and in underestimating the seriousness of the disorder.

At the moment it is very difficult to draw firm conclusions about the efficacies of different treatments. The challenge in the next few years is to accompany the setting up of services with careful evaluation of the alcoholic patients treated and their subsequent progress. Only by undertaking operational research of therapeutic services will more effective treatment of alcoholism be achieved.

Chapter 12

The Abstinent Alcoholic

Alcoholism is best regarded as a chronic disorder with a marked tendency towards relapse. This means that alcoholics remain vulnerable people even if they stop drinking. Prolonged management is therefore necessary. The 'cure' almost always, as we have discussed, calls for total abstinence from alcohol. In some respects they must continue to regard themselves as alcoholics, even though they have stopped drinking.

If there are serious physical complications from the alcoholism, it is all the more important that drinking must not be resumed. Even in the case of the inveterate chronic alcoholic it should be reduced as much as possible. Giving up alcohol improves the long-term survival of patients with liver cirrhosis. Sadly, abstinence proves inadequate to prevent the progression of liver disease in certain alcoholics, most often women, who are particularly susceptible to severe damage.

Abstinent alcoholics are found in many places. There are alcoholics in prison who are undergoing enforced sobriety; their drinking may have been the direct cause of their confinement, for imprisonment is the treatment meted out to a substantial proportion of alcoholics. They are abstinent under duress. The vast majority begin drinking as soon as they are released.

Alcoholics undergoing treatment in general hospitals are often untroubled by craving while they are confined to the ward. But the physician who concentrates on their liver disease or stomach ulcer may be lulled into unwarranted confidence that the drinking problem has been mastered, if, indeed, he or she is even aware of it. Almost invariably, however, the drinking will return when the patient leaves the hospital.

These alcoholics who are effectively prevented from drinking by their circumstances are not our principal concern in this chapter. We shall discuss those alcoholics who voluntarily become abstinent, deliberately, as a necessary means to prevent a relapse of their illness. Most of them will previously have been helped by one of the means outlined in Chapter 10.

Some alcoholics owe their abstinence to the programme of Alcoholics Anonymous. Abstinent AA members adhere to the Twelve Steps, reminding themselves always that they are 'powerless over alcohol' and will never be able to drink again. It is the famous twelfth step, carrying the message to other alcoholics, that brings about the activity which becomes the most meaningful in many members' lives. They help other alcoholics to recover by drawing on their personal experience and understanding; this gives purpose and value to lives which had seemed hopeless and pointless. Every successful AA member has the 'key to sobriety', and the responsibility and privilege to help fellow sufferers. With justifiable pride and pardonable error the fellowship proclaims that the 'world's best professionals' cannot help alcoholics to recover. The task falls upon AA members alone, the most strict of whom will not invoke the aid of physicians, ministers or social workers, although this absolutism is changing.

A number of medical clinics seek active collaboration with Alcoholics Anonymous; lack of staff may make this inevitable but a medical service which only advises AA attendance to outpatients is tacitly endorsing the AA claim that only the fellowship can keep alcoholics abstinent.

This is not so. Very many alcoholics who come to medical clinics have been to AA meetings but have not been able to derive benefit from the programme. It is not effective for every alcoholic or for every type of alcoholism. One of our patients put succinctly the objection that many feel: 'I tried AA for a year and found it a fascinating sociological phenomenon at first. But the masochistic bouts they indulged in over coffee appalled me, their re-living of their drunk-ups, getting up at meetings to purge themselves, the quality of evangelism I couldn't buy intellectually, and that turned me away finally, although I appreciated what it did for others.' Jellinek in his last book[57] pointedly warned: 'In spite of the respect and admiration to which Alcoholics Anonymous have a claim, on account of their great achievements, there is every reason why the student of alcoholism should not accept the exclusiveness of the picture of alcoholism as propounded by Alcoholics Anonymous.' Professional staff whose sole provision for the after-care of their patients is to recommend that they go to AA are remiss. Doctors, patients and relatives should be clearly aware that the fellowship works best with compulsive alcoholics in whom enduring craving for alcohol is prominent. These will find in AA one method for remaining abstinent and at the same time a social organization which can replace their harmful drinking associations.

The need to find new social contacts in place of former drinking relationships is sometimes the paramount problem for the abstinent alcoholic. Many never surmount it. Bacon[58] has analysed the stages by which membership of Alcoholics Anonymous enables abstinent drinkers to resume their place in society. First, they are dependent on a sponsor, who has twelve-stepped them during the faltering beginnings of sobriety. Then they become the confidant of the entire local group of alcoholics, hearing them confess publicly their own drinking history. In turn the alcoholic may become a sponsor and can aspire to a prominent place in the group. Bales[59] has indicated that the alcoholic by temperament prefers multiple personal relations with emphasis on emotional expression; in Alcoholics Anonymous intense, emotional associations of a very intimate sort come about between members who share each other's woes and triumphs. The concept of AA which alcoholics find immediately helpful is the view that they suffer not from weakness or depravity but from a disease; that it is a disease from which they can recover is proved by the abstinent alcoholics whom they get to know intimately.

Alcoholics Anonymous successes among the alcoholics studied by the Connecticut Commission were recognized as having achieved a spectacular shift in their lives.[60] Interviewers considered that these abstinent AA members had acquired a sense of purpose and value in life. In the process they had become 'as dependent on AA as they were on alcohol'. The interviewers also remarked, however, that many of the patients they studied had been unable to accommodate to the AA procedure.

The extension of National Health Service and other treatment facilities in Britain has enabled many people to stop drinking. These abstinent alcoholics need the continuing help of treatment services to consolidate their treatment gains. No service is functioning adequately unless serious help is given to the patients who are rehabilitating themselves socially. Responsible after-care is all the more important in the light of the finding that if an alcoholic remains abstinent for six months the future chances of continuing sobriety are very good.

The task facing recovered alcoholics is to stay off drink despite warm invitations by friends or gibes from the unsympathetic. In addition, they will have to combat without alcohol the tensions produced by sudden hazards in their daily lives, as well as those painful subjective feelings which are aroused by other people touching on vulnerable traits in their personality and exploiting, humiliating, angering or disappointing them. Even after months or years of abstinence the risk persists of recovered alcoholics again resorting to drinking and thus precipitating a rapid return of their former addictive pattern.

Although many abstinent alcoholics cherish the lingering hope that they may be able to revert to normal social drinking, such a happy outcome only very rarely occurs. Treated alcoholics who begin to drink again will almost certainly revert to their former drinking practices. Symptomatic excessive drinkers (see Chapter 7), of course, may after successful treatment of the underlying condition be able to drink again socially in a controlled way.

For many, the prospect of permanent abstinence is daunting. Alcoholics Anonymous recognizes and allows for this consternation by advocating that the abstinent alcoholic should think only about the next twenty-four hours, and resolve to negotiate only that stretch of time. Doctors who treat many alcoholics will have been chastened by the shudder and the pained look of reproof with which some alcoholics receive the information that they should never drink again. They prefer to plan only for the immediate future. Indeed for many this qualified resolve is the most realistic approach. If they have been modest in their undertaking they will not be completely demoralized by a relapse. We discussed in Chapter 10 the paradox that by omitting to take

Antabuse someone may resume drinking a few days later may help patients to agree to continue to take it. Abstinent alcoholics who do lapse can often learn from their failure by appreciating the sort of conflict situations which precipitate the recurrence of drinking.

The Spouse and Recovery

When an alcoholic is successfully treated and becomes abstinent this can materially alter the family equilibrium. A wife who has become used to making all the decisions and handling the finances of the family is not always ready to surrender these responsibilities to her spouse, though he is eager to resume them. Justifiably she fears that, if he relapses, then once again he will plunge them all into chaos from which they were slowly and painfully rescued by her own exertions and resourcefulness. So much she will be prepared to say to the doctor or social worker, but she will be far less ready to admit that she does not want to shed an authority in the family which was essential for survival.

If she allows him scope to take up some responsibilities she will have to stand by and watch him flounder ineptly as he endeavours, for instance, to exert discipline over his children, when for years past he has been in no position to try. Should she intervene she may well start him drinking again. This very point was well illustrated in the group discussion which we quoted in Chapter 10. The wife must be particularly careful in her attempts to help him with his treatment. If, for instance, he should be taking an Antabuse tablet each morning, she can support his resolve by approving his taking of it. In general, AA members insist that her best approach is not to watch over him but to leave him alone. Treatment staff, on the other hand, need to consider the conditions that apply in each case with regard to the personalities of the individual concerned.

Mostly, wives are pleased when their alcoholic husbands achieve abstinence. Life becomes richer for them. However, for some the abstinence of recovered spouses is difficult to bear because they become less active and socially more withdrawn.

Their circle of drinking friends may have been lost. A wife of an abstinent alcoholic may confess that she misses the gaiety of her husband's former drinking days. Now that he has recovered and she dares make comparisons again, he seems duller. Nevertheless, usually she is content to sit with him at home in the unaccustomed calm of his sobriety. She feels that the battle he has won has been a joint victory.

The spouse's peace of mind is never complete. All the time he or she knows that drinking may start again. Should the husband be late home the wife will begin to worry. If she cannot control her fears she may start phoning the office for news of him or even send out the children to go and look in the local public houses. When he returns he is dismayed by her unconcealed agitation and concern. He realizes that she is surreptitiously sniffing his breath, and her anxious regard signals to him that her trust in him is limited. Her anticipation of a relapse may actually precipitate one. Do we not all tend to fulfil the expectations others have for us?

A wife came to hospital with her husband when he began to drink again, after being abstinent for seven months. She interrupted the information she was providing to turn to him and say: 'I tried to reach you all afternoon. I had a knot in my stomach since half past five. I never moved from that window. My nails were down to the quick.' Panic-stricken waiting, the characteristic experience of the alcoholic's wife, had suddenly become a part of her existence once more.

Many a wife finds herself unprepared for the return of her husband's sexual potency. While he was drinking she had adjusted herself, first of all to intercourse being distasteful, then to its absence, which came as a relief. Now she has mixed feelings about his renewed sexual ardour. She may not welcome it yet she feels that to deny her husband will invite doubts and even jealousy to reassert themselves. A sympathetic psychiatric social worker can help the wife to express and examine these real difficulties and so work out what she must do.

The Adjustment of the Recovered Alcoholic

Abstinent alcoholics were studied by investigators working in the Commission on Alcoholism of the State of Connecticut.[61] In a group of 299 alcoholics, fifty-five were studied who had had uninterrupted abstinence for as long as a year. Giving up drinking was associated with general all-round improvement; they enjoyed improved health and better social, family and work relationships. The abstinent alcoholics looked better, felt better and viewed themselves as better people for being abstinent, and they were so regarded by others. But the investigators then undertook a closer examination into what they termed 'the nuances of their lives'. They classified the abstinent alcoholics into four sub-types. Half were overtly disturbed: for them abstinence was sustained in a setting of tension, anxiety, dissatisfaction or resentment. A quarter were called 'inconspicuously indequate': they showed what the interviewers rated as meagre involvement with life and living, and an absence of any marked sense of purpose, interest or excitement. A third group (12 per cent) were the successful AA members, who had achieved a sense of purpose and contentment through identification with the movement. A tenth of the abstinent alcoholics were named 'independent successes': they were self-respecting and seemed to have undergone personality growth with a resulting increased field of interest; they were not psychologically disturbed nor troubled by problems of resentment or aggression.

As this report makes clear, the alcoholics who had stopped drinking did not find things too easy. The achievement of sobriety does not always bring with it tranquillity of mind. They find that former friends are not as ready as they themselves are to believe that they have overcome their affliction. These friends are aware that the outlook for an alcoholic becoming 'cured' is not good, and therefore they react warily. Some, indeed, prefer to keep clear of the alcoholic, especially if in the past they have been let down or embarrassed. Though spouses generally return to or welcome back their partners when they have stopped drinking, former alcoholics may find it more difficult to reclaim a place in the affections of their children. The latter's feelings have often been bitterly hardened by the behaviour of the alcoholic during their most impressionable years.

Recovered alcoholics have to decide whether they are strong enough to tell new friends and new employers that they used to drink, knowing that if they do so they may find themselves condemned for it and their friendship repudiated. They will have to decide how to avoid having a drink when one is offered. Abstinent alcoholics are faced with numerous decisions which are all part of a large problem: should they try to return to the style of life they were attempting to lead when excessive drinking began, or should they start afresh on a new track? Former alcoholics resolve this dilemma each in their own way, but for all of them it is a crucial decision which has to be made, painfully and with difficulty. Because of this, treatment of alcoholics must aim at more than getting them to give up alcohol. It should endeavour to make them able to face the hazards of living that are still to come.

Chapter 13

Preventive Strategies and Public Health Aspects of Alcoholism

The World Health Assembly adopted a resolution (WHA 32.40) at its meeting in 1979 which states that 'problems related to alcohol, particularly its excessive consumption, rank among the world's major public health problems.' All governments have endorsed the serious concern it conveys.

In this chapter we present facts about the prevalence of alcoholism, its measurable harms and the extent of drinking. We go on to consider what might be done to prevent it and some of the moral and ethical dilemmas that arise if we seek to use measures to reduce the availability of alcohol. We go on to deal with such matters as down-and-out alcoholics and the links between alcoholism and crime. We discuss what further research is necessary and finally address the problem of how to get help.

The Prevalence of Alcoholism

The determination of the prevalence of alcoholism rests either upon identification, somehow, of alcoholics in the course of a population survey, or upon counting the number of people known to be suffering from an alcoholic harm. Clearly each of these is fraught with difficulty. Population surveys generally use a measure of drinking frequency and the quantity consumed. It can be readily appreciated that many do not own to the full extent of their drinking. Alternatively we can look to death rates from alcoholic causes, to numbers of admissions to general hospital wards or psychiatric units, to numbers detected by general practitioners (notorious for their understatements) and to figures of alcohol-related offences and any other harm that might be attributable to alcohol. Many alcoholics, of course, do not come to any agency interested in counting them.

Given the possibilities of error, it is not at all surprising that estimates vary. Quite surprisingly, however, they do not vary all that much. There is a large measure of agreement that there are somewhere upward of half a million alcoholics in the UK.

The Brewers Society, not a body inclined to overstate the numbers, has claimed that, of the 40 million drinkers in this country, 98 per cent drink moderately and suffer no problems.[62] Simple arithmetic tells us that the other 2 per cent amount to 800,000. The addition of those disadvantaged by an alcoholic in the home or by the bad work or absenteeism of a fellow employee, and those injured in accidents involving alcoholics, gives a much greater number who suffer the consequences of alcoholism. The Office of Health Economics[63] estimated that the number of heavy drinkers (without reference to their being harmed) was 3 million; 700,000 of these were classed as 'problem drinkers'; those physically dependent on alcohol were estimated at 150,000.

One method of quantifying drinking habits is the unit system; half a pint of beer, one glass of wine and one single measure of spirits are taken as equivalent quantities called one unit. The Royal College of Psychiatrists[64] used to consider that the daily consumption of eight units constituted a reasonable guideline for the upper limit of drinking. Using that yardstick, and allowing for a small measure of under-reporting (which such studies always show) and for the lower weights of women, a large and reliable recent survey[65] found that 6 per cent of men and 1 per cent of women were drinking above this level. In the 18–24 age group the figures were 13 per cent and 4 per cent. There was a considerable association between heavy drinking and those harms about which inquiry was possible. More recently, the Royal College of Psychiatrists have reduced their amounts that they consider may be drunk without risk of harm to twenty-one units per week for men and fourteen for women.[66]

A large Scottish survey[67] revealed that males more than females were regular drinkers. Most drinking was done by young adults, particularly men. This study claimed that 30 per cent of all the alcohol reported consumed was imbibed by a mere 3 per cent of those interviewed. Among all age groups and both sexes the unmarried were more often 'regular drinkers' than the married. Regular drinking in both men and women occurred more often in those who had friends who also drank regularly. The author of this study also reported an important minority of male drinkers (5 per cent) who expressed a desire to drink less. This proportion rises to 18 per cent among those men who acknowledge that they drink 'heavily' or 'quite a lot', compared with 13 per cent of those who actually do drink relatively heavily.

Consumption of alcohol has risen sharply since the Second World War. In 1950 it was estimated that in Britain we drank, on average, 3·7 litres of pure alcohol per head. In 1980 the corresponding figure was 7·8 litres – more than twice as much. The average yearly intake of those aged fifteen years or over is 240 pints of beer, twelve pints of cider, twenty-five pints of wine and nine pints of spirits. The cost of alcohol drunk in Britain is estimated as close to £20 billion a year.

Trends in choice of drink are shown on page 32. Although there has been a great increase in sales of wine and spirits relative to beer sales, beer still accounts for over half the alcohol imbibed in the United Kingdom; but among women more spirits and wines are consumed than beer, lager or cider. The heaviest drinkers are the youngest adults, those in their twenties.[68] Those most likely to be 'moderate' or 'heavy' drinkers are the young and single. Single men aged forty-five and over are heavier drinkers than their married male counterparts; this finding does not apply to women, where married and single middle-aged women drink similar quantities.

Life Expectancy

An established alcoholic who is not successfully treated has a greatly reduced expectation of life, and the official statistics of the Registrar General show that there is a greatly increased mortality rate among people in certain occupations (Table 1). Availability of alcohol at work has been held to attract people who already have a high level of alcohol consumption. Publicans, for instance, were found by one study[69] to have a death rate from cirrhosis of the liver nine times as high as for all men of comparable age.

Table 1 Liver cirrhosis mortality in England and Wales (1970–72)

Occupational groups	Standardized mortality ratio (all=100)
Publicans, innkeepers	1,576
Deck, engineering officers and pilots, ships	781
Barmen, barmaids	633
Fishermen	595
Proprietors and managers of boarding houses and hotels	506
Restaurateurs	385
Armed forces	367
Cooks	354
Authors, journalists and related workers	314
Medical practitioners	311
Tobacco preparers and product-makers	269

Source: Office of Population Censuses and Surveys

Cirrhosis deaths nearly doubled between 1970 and 1985 for both men and women.

David Cross, in a recent article,[70] reported that alcohol claimed 'up to 40,000 lives a year'. In the same article it was stated that 52 per cent of fire deaths and 45 per cent of fatal road accidents involving the young were linked to alcohol.

Rates of Admission for Treatment

We have earlier, when considering services, referred to the high proportions of alcoholic patients (especially men) admitted to general medical wards with an illness specifically related to alcoholism, and to the low rate of detection of their condition. Turning now to psychiatric units, including alcoholism treatment units, in 1975 there were about 13,500 admissions to National Health Service hospitals for treatment of alcoholism. In Great Britain as a whole between 1970 and 1977 total admissions to psychiatric hospitals for alcoholism and alcoholic psychosis increased by 74 per cent. Admissions for alcoholism represent a much larger proportion of total psychiatric admissions in Scotland (21 per cent in 1977) than in England and Wales (6·8 per cent). Alcoholism is commoner in Scotland, therefore, but a still higher first admission rate has been reported for Northern Ireland.

Preventive Measures

We have devoted a large section of this book to methods of treatment. Yet we live in an age that is rightly planning to devote more energy and resources to prevention, in the belief that this will lead to less morbidity. It is a belief we share. Thus, for instance, in Britain, the Department of Health and Social Security has issued two publications: *Prevention and Health: Everyone's business*[71] and *Drinking Sensibly*,[72] as well as the prevention report of its Advisory Committee on Alcoholism.[73] It is right for us, therefore, to discuss preventive strategies. We shall mostly be considering primary prevention, that is, stopping the development of the condition. We have not forgotten secondary and tertiary prevention, namely preventing worsening of the condition once it has developed and preventing relapse after recovery, but these have been dealt with in Chapter 10. Preventive measures must be preceded, of course, by recognition of the condition by the alcoholic and all those devoted to helping him or her. The patient also has to be persuaded to accept treatment.

For primary prevention we turn once more to the triad of host, agent and environment. In practical terms we cannot, simply to reduce alcoholism rates, provide a better environment for people. There are good general grounds for securing better housing, full employment and more stable marriages, but we cannot consider any of these to be desirable just so that fewer people should turn to alcohol to assuage their social distress.

It is possible to alter the host, that is to say, all of us, the people who might or might not become alcoholic, by way of education, and we shall deal with health education shortly.

We now consider measures aimed at the agent — at alcohol itself. These are all concerned with control of supply. The epidemiological data, which we have already summarized in Chapter 6, show without doubt that if the amount a community drinks is reduced there will be less alcoholism. We also know that it is possible for governments to take steps that result in a reduction of consumption. The question is, should such steps be taken? John Stuart Mill took an extreme view about this, holding that it was not a government's duty to restrict the choice of citizens for the sake of their health. People had the right, he claimed, to destroy themselves if they wished. He was, moreover, writing specifically in the context of alcohol and alcoholism. However, he produced a pragmatic solution. Since every government had the duty of raising taxes, these might as well be raised in a manner that benefited citizens' health!

The British Government raises very considerable taxation revenue from duties upon alcoholic drinks. Its reluctance to see measures taken to restrict supply, therefore, is understandable. On the other hand, if the government raised the level of duty upon alcohol they might, despite a reduction in sales, gain more money. But here other voices enter. The European Community, for instance, already considers that British levels of duty are too high, with a consequent loss of the chance of some countries to export more wine to Britain. But the overriding argument is this: Why should everybody's enjoyment of alcohol be eroded merely to save a minority of people from the consequences of their harmful drinking, when it is within their own power to avoid those consequences? We might be willing to pay more for lead-free petrol because the effects of lead fumes in the atmosphere cannot be avoided by anyone, including children, using the streets. In respect of alcohol, people have the choice. The freedom of the many, therefore, need not be sacrificed for the sake of the few, but just so long as the freedom does not become enticement.

There are other ways of controlling supply besides price control, although that is the most effective. Licensing laws govern the hours of permitted sale, the age below which youths may not be served and, through the licensing magistrates, the number of permitted outlets in any community. Each of these factors can be manipulated to make it easier or harder to get a drink. If permitted hours of sale are extended it will be good for tourism, good for the producers and good for anyone who wants more personal freedom. However, since publicans will not keep open longer unless more drink is sold, at least sufficient to cover their increased wages bill, the effect of liberalizing hours of permitted sale will be to increase consumption and consequently, as we now know, the number of alcoholics. Were those responsible for extending pub opening hours aware of this?

Scotland obtained new licensing laws as a result of recommendations made by the Departmental Committee on Scottish Licensing Law. Since December 1976 bars have been open until 11 p.m., closing time being an hour later than formerly. Sunday licences, which were not previously allowed, have been issued for public houses since October 1977. Hopes appear to have been justified.[74] The rate of drinking seems to have become slower with the provision of the extra hour. Pressure to drink a lot rapidly seems reduced.

However, the reduced drinking rate in Scotland may have been effected by reasons other than the liberalization of licensing hours, so caution is appropriate in drawing firm conclusions. New laws passed in Finland in 1969 to make alcohol more readily accessible resulted in increased drinking at all levels of intake, particularly the rate of heavy use.[75]

Similar considerations apply to numbers of outlets. In Chapter 4 we referred to the recent rise in supermarket outlets. We have no wish to suppress any of these developments; however, we do want them to be determined by people who are aware of the public health implications.

One means of control that has not been used in Britain is to make it an offence for publicans to sell alcohol to anyone whom they consider to be already the worse for drink, or who is a known alcoholic. Regulations of this sort exist in the Federal Republic of Germany and are said to be liked by publicans as it gives them a means of control of the atmosphere of their establishments. Whether such a move would be popular in Britain we cannot say. It deserves to be considered.

It is always difficult to calculate the effect that any single measure relating to availability of supply may have upon the extent of alcoholism, because other factors, such as price and educational campaigns and the development of treatment services, are changing at the same time. That is why we refuse to line up with the Jeremiahs who see every step designed to make drinking more available and pleasurable or to make drink itself easier to come by as a step on an inexorable slope towards more alcoholism.

Health Education

We must attempt to educate about alcohol and its effects, both good and bad. Such education should deal with the effects upon the body and psychological changes brought on by alcohol, the state of drunkenness, reasonable limits of quantity and frequency of drinking and the special hazards in relation to driving. People must also be taught how to recognize signs of excessive drinking and alcoholism in themselves and in others, where help can be obtained and about the benefit of getting help.

The Health Education Council spends some three quarters of a million pounds a year on such education. This has to be set against the huge expenditure by the drink trade on advertising. The work of the HEC is hampered because schoolchildren are not taught, as part of the core curriculum, anything about how their bodies work: what the liver, for example, is and does. It is true to say that British children today are likely to be taught more about the body politic than about the body. Consequently they have no basis of fact upon which to hang educational messages about the effects of alcohol. The HEC has conducted media campaigns for many years now. These have not been subjected to any worthwhile evaluation, so we do not know to what extent they have been effective (though this will not be true of its current programmes centred on the south-west and the north-west health regions of England).

We believe that people are educable and we therefore follow the Department of Health and Social Security in regarding health education as a mainstay in preventing alcoholism. We would like to see the production of educational material suitable for use by general practitioners, health visitors and district nurses. These are the front-line troops of health education for adults, just as school teachers are for the young.

Educational measures have to counter adverse and harmful cultural attitudes. It is still regarded as manly to drink and to be able to hold one's liquor. Abstinent people, on the other hand, are regarded as weak. Indeed, this is one of the fears that alcoholics often voice when they are told they should become abstinent: 'How can I face my friends?' Cultural attitudes die hard, but that is no reason why they should not be tackled. Is it necessary for so many characters in films, plays and television dramas to be seen drinking, even when this forms no necessary part of the action? Subtly these pieces, which the producers would call verismo, work their effects. If he, why not I? If she, why not I?

Safe Limits

Most health educators nowadays like to give an indication of what are safe limits for drinking. We are not altogether persuaded of the virtue of this, because different people have different susceptibilities to the effects of alcohol. Also, these limits are often stated without saying safe for what – for driving, or to cause no impairment of health. Moreover, bodies such as the Royal College of Psychiatrists proclaim different safe limits at different times. Nevertheless, we feel obliged to offer their recommendations. Using the unit system of counting drinks, one unit is equivalent to half a pint of beer or a glass of wine or a single measure of spirits. The Royal College now advocates not more, on a regular basis, than twenty-one units per week for a man and fourteen units a week for a woman.

Advertising

Advertising of drinks works counter to health education. It is a massive industry, spending many millions of pounds annually in Britain, and subject to little statutory control. Voluntary agreements between advertisers and the TV companies have seen to it that drinks are not advertised until after children are supposed to be (but frequently are not) in bed. Moreover, no advertising of drink in Britain is allowed to glamorize drinking or indicate that sexual prowess is gained by drinking. Interpretation of this is, we may say, liberal to a degree.

Advertisers claim that all that advertising does is to cause brand switching. We doubt this and certainly we have seen some evidence that it affects total sales.

Some people have urged that drink advertisements, and indeed bottles of drink, should carry government health warnings similar to those on cigarette packets. We cannot agree because, whereas smoking is never beneficial, we believe that social drinking ought not to be represented as damaging.

Drunken Driving

Road accidents are among the most prominent and serious social consequences of drinking. The effect of alcohol upon driving performance has been extensively studied: there is progressive impairment of skill, judgement and reaction time from the first drink onwards. The drinkers themselves become progressively less able to detect their own impairment. Apart from the decline in driving performance, the same release of inhibitions which forms the social reason for drinking will affect drinkers' driving styles. They might not remain content to stay behind another car but will strive to overtake, often dangerously. Why give way to avoid an accident? Let the other driver do it. Too bad if they have also had a drink and feel the same. In Britain the peak rate for road accidents coincides with the hour after the pubs close, when an army of incapables is loosed on to the roads. In a survey of 2,000 road accidents, a drinking driver was involved in 25 per cent, and his or her condition was judged to be a major factor in 9 per cent. Drunken pedestrians also present a hazard. In one study, every one of a group of sixty-four pedestrians admitted to a Manchester hospital between midnight and 6 a.m. after being injured in a road accident was intoxicated.[76] It is reasonable to suppose that those who were killed were in like state. But drunken drivers cause most harm. The importance of a high blood alcohol concentration in drivers as a major factor in causing road accidents has been demonstrated many times. Large numbers of accidents, involving large numbers of injuries and deaths, could be prevented annually in Britain if drivers and pedestrians did not go on the roads after drinking.

Of course, drunken drivers are not necessarily alcoholics. Indeed, the view has often been put forward that alcoholics are relatively harmless on the roads because they render themselves incapable of driving a car at all. Recently, however, incontrovertible evidence has been produced showing that alcoholics do get into trouble for drunken driving. The majority of alcohol-related crashes are not caused by drunken drivers who exceed the blood alcohol level once in a while, but by persistent drinkers. An investigation of 2,000 persons arrested in Philadelphia for drunken driving demonstrated that 64 per cent could clearly be diagnosed as alcoholic.[77] A study of fatally injured drivers in Canada showed that 47 per cent had been drinking, and of these 80 per cent had extremely high blood alcohol levels.[78]

The increase in road accidents on the part of young males has been considered largely the result of more drinking at an increasingly young age. Drinking and driving is one of the commonest causes of death among male drivers in their twenties in the United Kingdom. Forty-five per cent of those killed had blood alcohol levels over the legal limit.[79]

In 1967 legislation came into force in Britain making it an offence, with automatic revocation of licence, to drive with an alcohol concentration of more than 80 milligrams in 100 millilitres of blood. The blood alcohol test has now been replaced by a breath alcohol measurement carried out by police (35 micrograms in 100 millilitres is the limit). It is an offence to refuse to be tested.

The permitted levels would ordinarily be exceeded by drinking ten single whiskies or five pints of beer. Few authorities are happy about such a high figure, and most believe that a concentration of 50 milligrams per 100 millilitres is the highest that could be accepted as consistent with safe driving. Despite these limits it is not uncommon for those tested to produce levels two, three, four or more times as high. Between one third and one half of the fatal road accidents occur in adults with excessive alcohol (and/or other drug) blood levels.[80]

In the twenty years since the introduction of the legislation, 1·1 million motorists have been found guilty of drink-driving offences. However, it still remains that only 13 per cent of drivers involved in accidents are breathalysed. Blood and breath tests have considerably reduced drunken driving accident rates, but more could be prevented if the police were permitted to do random testing instead of having to show good reason before stopping a driver. Such a move is still being firmly resisted by the Government.

The evidence that a substantial proportion of those involved in drunken-driving offences are alcoholics should suggest to the authorities an additional profitable approach. This would be to institute a programme of routine evaluation of the alcoholism status of those brought before the Courts and the offering of proper treatment facilities when appropriate. This could be coupled with a refusal to reissue drivers with a licence until they could demonstrate that they had received treatment and reduced their drinking.

Skid Rows

In all cities there are areas where down-and-out alcoholics gather. The Bowery in New York is perhaps the best known of these 'skid rows', a term that somehow indicates the slippery slope down which these alcoholics have fallen. Respectable citizens may not know the site of the skid row in their particular cities, but the police are in no doubt. These areas are characteristically where the cheapest lodging-houses are to be found. Down-and-out alcoholics spend the day in warm places such as stations, if they are not moved out into the streets, and the night, if they are lucky, in a lodging-house. If not, they sleep under bridges or on derelict sites, where there is the company of fellows in the same state. Some clergymen offer such alcoholics nightly shelter in church crypts. Many of these people are methylated spirits drinkers. They present a serious problem to the communities in which they live.

In skid row the alcoholic finds two desirable things: anonymity and the absence of society's strictures against drinking excesses. Alcoholics do not get to skid row from choice, but once there they may appreciate what it offers them. This is the chance to abandon themselves to drinking, immune from the shame resulting from the criticism of people who object, and relatively unmolested by the police. These areas are eyesores and a matter for distress to the civic-minded. Nevertheless, they serve a purpose for society by providing a retreat for those who extruded themselves when they gave up the struggle to remain socialized. Skid rows perform a function in the cities which generate them.

From any point of view, skid row presents an important public health problem. Homeless, indigent and sometimes destitute people die there from the consequences of alcoholism. But even without this, since we now look upon alcoholism as an illness, these areas constitute reservoirs of ill people, in which affected people sink steadily and to which newcomers are constantly drifting. Skid rows cannot be dealt with by cleaning up the neighbourhood. Unless a more satisfactory solution is found for the individuals concerned, the problem has not been tackled. Hostels are required, with sheltered workshops and energetic social welfare measures that might enable these people to return by degrees to health and self-respect. Without this, there is no hope.

Most communities do more than just tacitly provide a skid row area in their town. For alcoholics who will not make use of treatment services, for alcoholics who are irrecoverable, they provide some charity and care. This is generally through support for organizations which accept the challenge of helping seemingly hopeless cases, particularly those who are homeless and jobless. In Britain the Salvation Army, its officers and its hostels have eased the existence of innumerable deteriorating alcoholics.

The Salvation Army has been impelled to enter the field of treatment as well. In a few places special homes have been set up where alcoholics are accepted who show 'a sincere personal longing for deliverance'. What began as a charitable concern for the destitute, based on religious precept, still remains so. But the workers have learned that care and charity by themselves are not enough; they have evolved a treatment orientation.

Alcohol and Crime

Another measure which the community adopts to deal with alcoholics is *imprisonment*. Drunkenness is not itself an offence in Britain, though people are still charged with being 'drunk and incapable' or 'drunk and disorderly'. Alcoholics are also picked up by the police for loitering and for vagrancy. First offenders get small fines for such offences, but when they are often repeated magistrates send people to prison. Alcoholics are to be found in large numbers in most jails. Some alcoholics regard prison as a place of refuge. Food and shelter are provided there, devoid of any moralizing, which they feel they get from the Salvation Army, and without their being considered as mad, which is the impression they sometimes receive in psychiatric hospitals.

A study of long-term recidivist prisoners in London found that 11 per cent were severely dependent on alcohol and serving sentences for drunkenness, while another 19 per cent were severely dependent and imprisoned for non-drunkenness offences.[81]

Alcoholics were thought to have little wish to be treated and to look on the condition as wrong behaviour rather than illness. Prison alcoholics were considered to have little motivation for treatment even if it was offered to them. Views have changed, and it has been urged that more therapeutic units such as the one for treating alcoholics at Wormwood Scrubs should be set up. Imprisonment is quite ineffective as a treatment for alcoholism. Alternative approaches will have to be devised if the community wishes these people to be helped. It is important to recognize that, although alcoholics in prison may also have served sentences for offences other than drunkenness, such offences are usually a thing of the past. Prison alcoholics are commonly committed because of their abnormal use of alcohol rather than for any palpably criminal behaviour.

The recommendation has been made that the traditional penal approach should be replaced by care and rehabilitation, with detoxification centres set up to which drunken people can be taken, instead of locking them up in the police cells.[82] The Department of Health and Social Security issued a circular in 1973 on community services for alcoholics. These laudable reforms still have far to go.

Detoxification centres, however, whatever their achievement in helping alcoholics to become sober, do not manage to persuade alcoholics into treatment programmes. They are an alternative to the cells, but not one which many drunken offenders prefer. Indeed, the detoxification centres have proved more effective with medical than with police referrals.

While our concern in this book has been alcoholics who are capable of recognizing their need for treatment and of responding to it, we do not want the responsibility of the community towards the more deteriorated alcoholic to be overlooked. We hope that, as treatment services become more adequate, fewer alcoholics will deteriorate to levels of helplessness. At present the need is to provide alcoholics themselves with an understanding of possible paths to recovery, and to serve upon responsible authorities most definite intimation that the proper place for alcoholics, however deteriorated they may be, is neither the gutter nor the jail.

What is needed are places simply equipped and staffed, where drunken people may go for sobering up. While there, some of them may welcome an assessment of their physical and social status and helpful advice as to how their needs in these areas may be met. A few of them may even be persuaded into treatment programmes. All of them would receive shelter, care, food and warmth. It is not much to expect a civilized community to make such provision available.

What must not be done is to take away the present police role and leave drunkenness offenders in the gutter. We fear this might happen if decriminalization was introduced without adequate alternative provision being made.

Research

A great deal of research is still required before many of the fundamental questions of alcoholism are solved. Research will have to be carried out in many different areas — biochemistry, pharmacology, clinical medicine, sociology and public health. We list the most important areas of possible research. The studies we indicate are called for to provide answers to questions which arise in clinical practice.

Biochemical and Physiological Research

Studies to explore the body changes that take place in response to prolonged drinking.

Studies of alterations in the body's response to alcohol. Why are some people more prone than others to get withdrawal symptoms? What is the mechanism whereby tolerance at first increases in alcoholics and later decreases?

Would reducing the alcohol strength of drinks, particularly spirits, result in less alcohol being consumed or merely in more volume being drunk?

Clinical Studies

Investigation of the course of alcoholism in the young. The personality characteristics of alcoholics, especially the identification of patterns of behaviour which were present before the excessive drinking. What changes in personality are produced by the alcoholism itself?

Determination of the sub-types of alcoholism. Statistical studies of the course and outcome of the different varieties of alcoholism.

Stages in recovery from alcoholism. Why do some abstinent alcoholics adjust well while others remain poorly adjusted?

What is the incidence of physical illnesses attributable to alcoholism?

How frequent are the brain diseases attributable to alcoholism?

The investigation of alcoholism in women.

A systematic study of the effect of alcoholics on their families.

Preventive Measures

The identification of pre-alcoholism, so as to be able to advise and protect vulnerable individuals before alcoholic harms develop.

The investigation of measures which will make excessive drinkers come forward for evaluation and treatment.

Whether an information service makes members of the community more understanding of, and helpful towards, alcoholics.

What measures can be developed to influence social agencies (governmental, local authority and voluntary) to adopt a more effective approach to alcoholics?

What are the effects of manipulating social controls – price, licensing, taxation, hours of permitted sale – on the incidence of both drunkenness and alcoholism?

What proportion of persons convicted of drunkenness are alcoholic? What proportion of those involved in drunken driving accidents are alcoholic? What effect would routine police tests of drivers involved in accidents and, for those convicted, stiffer penalties such as imprisonment, have on reduced drunken driving?

Social and Cultural Factors

The study of the form and relative prevalence of alcoholism in different cultures and in different groups (e.g. ethnic, religious and social class) within a single culture. These studies would be concerned with the prevalence of alcoholism within the various groups, the forms which it takes and the actions taken by the alcoholics themselves, their families and their social group to deal with the problem.

Estimation of the economic cost of alcoholism. There is the cost of medical services, and the cost of accidents, but there are also hidden costs which may well amount to a great sum. The cost of absenteeism, the loss to firms of key personnel who become incapacitated at the height of their working powers, the cost of provision of children's care services, the cost to the social services of supporting the family.

Treatment Studies

Comparison of different methods of treatment for alcoholism.

What are the success rates of the different methods of treatment?

How To Get Help

The system of medical services is familiar to most citizens. It involves, as the point of first contact, the general practitioner or family physician, either coming on a home visit or at the health centre. However, for many alcoholics the first point of medical contact is the accident and emergency department of a hospital. This can arise because of an accident or illness often associated with intoxication, but another reason is that the alcoholic may not be registered with a family doctor, or else not with one near at hand.

Alcoholics who view doctors as authority figures likely to be critical, judgemental or condemnatory, may prefer to turn first to other helpers.

Social workers may be the first professionals who are involved. In the majority of such instances the distress of the spouse or children may have been the reason for the contact.

Apart from these statutory professional workers, a network of voluntary helping agencies exists. If alcoholics think they will be best understood by others like them, they will naturally turn to Alcoholics Anonymous, and they can find the address of a local branch in the telephone directory. In most areas of the United Kingdom there are local councils on alcoholism, also listed in the phone directory, and the people to be met there are skilled in giving help and in directing alcoholics towards more expert help. Many of these councils are glad to welcome alcoholics who simply walk into their premises. The Salvation Army is equally welcoming and runs several hostels for alcoholics.

All these agencies, both statutory and voluntary, and including also the alcoholism treatment units and community psychiatric nursing services, ought to work together harmoniously to provide an interlocking network of services. We have to say that this is not always the case, and deplore the jealousies and rivalries that exist. Alcohol Concern, largely dependent on government funding, aims both to help integrate services and to act as a lobby for their improvement. The Medical Council on Alcoholism preserves its independence from Alcohol Concern and aims at the education of doctors and the promotion of medical research into alcoholism.

We mention all these agencies and bodies to assist an alcoholic in getting help, and to emphasize the large number of people willing to provide it.

Notes

1. World Health Organization (1952). *Alcohol Subcommittee Second Report.* WHO Technical Reports Series, no. 48.
2. Cohen, J., Dearnaley E. J., and Hansel, C. E. M. (1958). 'The risk taken in driving under the influence of alcohol'. *British Medical Journal*, i. 1438.
3. Kessel, N., and Grossman, G. (1961). 'Suicide in alcoholics'. *British Medical Journal*, ii, 1671.
4. Norvig, J., and Neilsen, B. (1956). 'A follow-up study of 221 alcohol addicts in Denmark'. *Quarterly Journal of Studies on Alcohol*, 17, 663.
5. Robinson, A., Platt, S., Foster, J., and Kreitman, N. (1987). 'Report on parasuicide in Edinburgh'. Medical Research Council Unit for Epidemiological Studies in Psychiatry.
6. Jones, K. L., and Smith, D. W. (1975). 'The fetal alcohol syndrome'. *Teratology*, 12, 1.
7. Kaminski, M., Rumeau-Rouquette, C. Schwartz, D. (1976). 'Consommation d'alcool chez les femmes enceintes et issue de la grossesse'. *Revue d'Epidémiologie, Médecine Sociale et Santé Publique*, 24, 27–40.
8. Kessel, N., and Woolf, P. S. Unpublished study.
9. Horton, D. (1943). 'The function of alcohol in primitive societies: A crosscultural study'. *Quarterly Journal of Studies on Alcohol*, 4, 199.
10. Wilson, P. (1980). 'Drinking in England and Wales'. *Population Trends 1980.* London: HMSO.
11. Seebohm Rowntree, B., and Lavers, G. R. (1951). *English Life and Leisure.* London: Longmans.
12. Skolnick, J. H. (1957). 'The stumbling block'. Doctoral dissertation, Yale University.
13. Makela, K. (1972). 'Consumption level and cultural drinking patterns as determinants of alcohol problems'. Amsterdam: 30th International Congress on Alcoholism and Drug Dependence.
14. Trevelyan, G. M. (1944). *English Social History.* London: Longmans Quoted by permission of the publishers.
15. Trevelyan, G. M., op. cit.
16. Vaillant, G. E. (1982) 'Natural history of male alcoholism'. *Journal of Studies on Alcohol*, 43, 216.
17. Jellinek, E. M. (1960). *The Disease Concept of Alcoholism.* New Haven: Hillhouse Press.
18. Edwards, G., and Grant, M. (eds.) (1977). *Alcoholism: New knowledge and new responses.* London: Croom Helm.
19. Orford, J., Oppenheim, E., Egbert, S., Hemsman, C., and Guthrie, S. (1976).

'The cohesiveness of alcohol-complicated marriages and its influence on treatment outcome'. *British Journal of Psychiatry*, 128, 318.

20. Kaufman, E., and Kaufman, P. (eds) (1979). *Family Therapy of Drug and Alcohol Abuse*. New York: Gardner.

21. Finney, J. W., Moos, R. H., and Mewborn, C. R. (1980). 'Post-treatment experiences and treatment outcome of alcoholic parents six months and two years after hospitalization'. *Journal of Consulting and Clinical Psychology*, 48, 17.

22. Aronson, H., and Gilbert, A. (1963). 'Pre-adolescent sons of male alcoholics'. *Archives of General Psychology*, 8, 235.

23. Nylander, I. (1960). 'The children of alcoholic fathers'. *Acta Paediatrica Scandinavica*, 49, supplement 121.

24. Aronson, H., and Gilbert, A., op. cit.

25. Keane, A., and Roche, D. (1974). 'Developmental disorders in the children of male alcoholics'. Proceedings of the 20th International Institute on the Prevention and Treatment of Alcoholism, Manchester, England.

26. Cork, R. M. (1969). *The Forgotten Children*. Toronto: Addiction Research Foundation.

27. Wilkins, R. H. (1974). *The Hidden Alcoholic in General Practice*. London: Elek.

28. Owens, E. P. (1981). 'Prevalence of alcoholism among men admitted to general medical wards'. Paper presented to the epidemiology section of the International Congress of Alcohol Addiction, Vienna.

29. Jariwalla, A. G., Adams, P. H., and Hore, B. D. (1979). 'Alcohol and acute general medical admissions to hospital'. *Health Trends*, 11, 95.

30. Jarman, C. M. B., and Kellett, J. M. (1979). 'Detecting excessive drinking among admissions to a general hospital'. *British Medical Journal*, 2, 469.

31. Barrison I. G., Viola, L., and Murray-Lyon, I. M. (1980). 'Do housemen take an adequate drinking history?'. *British Medical Journal*, 281, 1040.

32. Department of Health and Social Security (1987). *Alcohol Related Problems in Higher Professional and Postgraduate Medical Education*. London: DHSS.

33. Kessel. N., Hore, B. D., Makenjuola, J. D. A., Redmond, A. D., Rossall, C. J., Rees, D. W., Chand, T. G., Gordon, M., and Wallace, P. C. (1984). 'The Manchester detoxification service: Description and evaluation'. *Lancet*, i, 839.

34. Kessel, N., *et al.* (1984), op. cit.

35. Silkworth, W. D. (1937). 'Alcoholism as a manifestation of allergy'. *Medical Record*, 145, 249.

36. Alcoholics Anonymous (1963). 'The Bill W. – Carl Jung letters'. Grapevine, January, 26.

37. Denzin, N. K. (1987). *The Alcoholic Self*. London and California: Sage.

38. Jellinek, E. M., op. cit.

39. Maxwell, M. A. (1962). 'Alcoholics Anonymous: An interpretation'. In Pitt-

man, D. J., and Snyder, C. R (eds), *Society, Culture and Drinking Patterns*. New York: Wiley.

40. Lemere, F., and Voegtlin, W. L. (1950). 'An evaluation of the aversion treatment of alcoholism'. *Quarterly Journal of Studies on Alcohol*, 8, 261.

41. Pattison, E. M. (1968). 'A critique of alcohol treatment concepts: with special reference to abstinence'. *Quarterly Journal of Studies on Alcohol*, 27, 49.

42. Davies, D. L., Shepherd, M., and Myers, E. (1956). 'The two-year prognosis of 50 alcoholic addicts after treatment in hospital'. *Quarterly Journal of Studies on Alcohol*, 17, 485.

43. Glatt, M. M. (1959). 'An alcoholic unit in a mental hospital'. *Lancet*, ii. 397.

44. Costello, R. M. (1975a). 'Alcoholism treatment and evaluation'. *International Journal of Addiction*, 10, 251.

45. Costello, R. M. (1975b). 'Alcoholism treatment and evaluation: Collation of two-year follow-up studies'. *International Journal of Addiction*, 10, 857.

46. Emrick, C. D. (1974). 'A review of psychologically oriented treatment of alcoholism: I. The use and interrelationship of outcome criteria and drinking behaviour following treatment'. *Quarterly Journal of Studies on Alcohol*, 35, 523; and Emrick, C. D. (1975). 'A review of psychologically oriented treatment of alcoholism: II. The relative effectiveness of different treatment approaches and the effectiveness of treatment versus no treatment'. *Quarterly Journal of Studies on Alcohol*, APC volume.

47. Selzer, M. L., and Holloway, W. H. (1957). 'A follow-up of alcoholics committed to state hospital'. *Quarterly Journal of Studies on Alcohol*, 18, 98.

48. Emrick, C. D. (1974), op cit.

49. Davies, D. L. (1962). 'Normal drinking in recovered alcoholics'. *Quarterly Journal of Studies on Alcohol*, 23, 94.

50. Armor, D. J., Polich, J. M., and Stambul, H. B. (1978). *Alcoholism and Treatment*. New York: Wiley.

51. Sobell, M. B., and Sobell, L. C. (1978). *Behavioral Treatment of Alcohol Problems: Individualized therapy and controlled drinking*. New York: Plenum.

52. Caddy, G. R., Addington, H. J., and Perkins, D. (1978). 'Individualized behaviour therapy for alcoholics: A third-year independent double-blind follow-up'. *Behavioral Research and Therapy*, 16, 345.

53. Pendery, M. L., Maltzman, I. M., and West. L. J. (1982). 'Controlled drinking by alcoholics: New findings and a re-evaluation of a major affirmative study'. *Science*, 217, 169.

54. Costello, R. M. (1975a), op. cit.

55. Orford, J., and Edwards, G. (1977). *Alcoholism: A comparison of treatment and advice*. London: Oxford University Press.

56. Chick, J., Ritson, B., Connaughton, J., and Stewart, A. (1988). 'Advice versus extended treatment for alcoholism: A controlled study'. *British Journal of Addiction*, 83, 159.

57. Jellinek, E. M., op. cit.

58. Bacon, S. D. (1957). 'A sociologist looks at Alcoholics Anonymous'. *Minnesota Welfare*, 10, 35.

59. Bales, R. F. (1942). 'Types of social structure as factors in "cures" for alcoholic addiction'. *Applied Anthropology*, 1, 1.

60. Gerard, D. L., Saenger, G., and Wile, R. (1962). 'The abstinent alcoholic'. *Archives of General Psychiatry*, 6, 83.

61. Gerard, D. L., *et al.*, op. cit.

62. The Brewers Society (1981). *A Strategy for the Prevention of Problem Drinking*. London: Arch Press.

63. Office of Health Economics (1981). *Alcohol: Reducing the harm*. Luton: White Crescent Press.

64. Royal College of Psychiatrists (1979). *Alcohol and Alcoholism*. London: Tavistock Publications.

65. Wilson, P. (1980). *Drinking in England and Wales*. London: HMSO.

66. Royal College of Psychiatrists (1986). *Alcohol: Our favourite drug*. London: Tavistock Publications.

67. Dight, S. (1976). *Scottish Drinking Habits*. London: HMSO.

68. Plant, M. A., (1982). *Drinking and Problem Drinking*. London: Junction Books.

69. Plant, M. A. (1982), op. cit.

70. Cross, D. (1987). *The Times*, 9 October 1987.

71. Department of Health and Social Security (1976). *Prevention and Health: Everyone's business*. London: HMSO.

72. Department of Health and Social Security (1981). *Drinking Sensibly*. London: HMSO.

73. DHSS Advisory Committee on Alcoholism (1977). *Report on Prevention*. London: HMSO.

74. Knight, I., and Wilson P. (1980). *Scottish Licensing Hours*. London: Office of Population Censuses and Surveys, HMSO.

75. Kiviranta, P. (1974). *Alcoholism Syndrome in Finland*. Helsinki: Finnish Foundation for Alcohol Studies.

76. Cassie, A. B., and Allan, W. R. (1961). 'Alcohol and road traffic accidents'. *British Medical Journal*, ii, 1668.

77. Fine, E. W., and Scoles, P. (1976). In Seixas, F. A., and Eggleston, S. (eds), *Work in Progress on Alcoholism*. New York: Annals of the New York Academy of Sciences, vol. 273.

78. Simpson, H. M., Warren, R. A., Page-Valin, L., and Collard, D. (1978) *Analysis of Fatal Traffic Crashes in Canada*. Ottawa: Traffic Injury Research Foundation of Canada.

79. Organization for Economic Cooperation and Development (1978). *New Research on the Role of Alcohol and Drugs in Road Accidents*. Paris: OECD.

80. Department of the Environment (1976). *Drinking and Driving: Report of the departmental committee (Blenner Lassett Committee)*. London: HMSO.

81. Edwards, G., Hensman, C., and Peto, J. (1971). 'Drinking problems among recidivist prisoners'. *Psychological Medicine*, 1, 388.
82. Home Office Committee on Treatment of the Chronic Drunkenness Offender within the Penal System, 1971.

Index

absenteeism, x, 5, 85, 88, 169
Abstem, 111–15
abstinence
  adjustment to, 151–2
  aim of treatment, 108–9, 131, 138,
    141–4, 145
  of compulsive alcoholics, 74, 75
  dry periods, 90
  inability to achieve, 73
  involuntary, 138, 145
  popular view of, ix, 161
  problems with, 72
  temporary, 4
  therapy, after, 119–21
  total, 2, 35, 145, 148
  voluntary, 161
  see also remission; withdrawal
    symptoms
Accept (voluntary agency), 134
acetaldehyde, 111–12
addicts, alcohol, 2
advertising, 160, 161–2
age of drinkers, 37, 60, 64, 158, 163,
  168
aggression; see violence
alcohol
  as cause of alcoholism, 57–9
  effects of, 9–12
  lack of training in medical schools,
    108
  nature of, 7–8
Alcohol Concern, 170
alcohol-related disabilities, 6
Alcoholics Anonymous (AA)
  allergy factor, and, 62, 130–31
  chronic alcoholics, 92
  compulsive alcoholics, 70, 75, 147
  formation of, 34, 130
  programme of, 131–4
  success of, 151

  treatment by, 106, 136, 146–9,
    170
allergies, 62, 130–31
American Medical Association, 5
amnesia, 20–22, 75, 83–5, 91
anaemia, 15, 116
anger, 11, 53
  see also violence
anorexia, 13
Antabuse, 111–15, 139, 143, 149
aphrodisiac, alcohol as, 9
apomorphine, 134–5
Armor, D. J, 142
assessments of alcoholics
  efficacy of, 143
  examinations prior to, 6, 109
  medical or social problem, 6
  prior to treatment, 109
availability of drink, 29–34, 58–61,
  64, 153, 157–60
aversion treatment, 134–5

Bacon, S. D., 147
Bales, R. F., 147
Barrison, I. G., 107
bars; see public houses
beer, 7, 155
black outs; see amnesia
blood
  alcohol in, 11–12
  red cells, changes in, 15
bodily damage; see harm, physical
bout drinkers, 78–9
brain
  amnesia, 85
  cells, destruction of, 22
  delirium tremens, 19
  disease, alcoholism as symptom of,
    77–8

effect of alcohol on, 10–11, 62–3,
    126, 168
epilepsy, alcoholic, 20
scanning, 22, 62
tolerance levels of, 12
treatment of, 116
breathalysers, 9, 163–4
Brewers Society, 34, 154

calories in alcohol, 9, 13
causes of alcoholism, 57–69
Chick, J., 143
children of alcoholics, 103–5,
    120–21, 149, 151–2, 169
    see also families; parents
chlordiazepoxide, 111
chlormethiazole, 111
chronic alcoholism, 3, 14, 80–81,
    91–2, 139, 145
chronic intoxication, 56
cider, 7–8
cirrhosis; see liver
citrated calcium carbimide, 111–15
classification of drinkers, 3
community psychiatric nurses, 123,
    170
compulsive alcoholics, 70, 74–6, 147
confabulation, 21
Connecticut Commission, 147, 151
consumption of alcohol, 1, 30–34,
    155, 159
cost (economic) of alcoholism, 169
Costello, R. M., 139–40
courts, unsuitability of, 5
crime
    alcoholism as, 59, 127–8, 166
    caused by alcohol, x, 42, 153
Cross, David, 156
custodial sentences; see prison

Davies, D. L., 139, 141–2
definition of alcoholism, 1–6
'degrees proof', 8
dehydration, 16
delirium tremens, 17–20, 24, 72, 92
dementia, 22

denial, 45
dependence
    alcoholic, 2, 3–4, 17, 83–91:
        compulsive alcoholics, of, 75;
        morbid, 41; neurotic alcoholics,
        of, 76; pregnancy, in, 27; stage
        in alcoholism, as, 80–81;
        syndrome, 3; unsuspected,
        70–72; vicious circle of, 65–6
    of alcoholics on others, 42–4, 48–9
depravity of temperament, 57
depression, 11, 76–8
detoxification, 110–11, 127, 136
    centres, 128–9, 166–7
diabetes, 15
diagnosis of alcoholism, 19, 71
    see also doctors; illness
diet
    cause of alcoholism, as, 62
    deficiency of, 13–14, 72
    improvement of, 116
dipsomania, 78–9
disorientation, 17–18
distillation, 8
disulfiram, 111–15
divorce; see spouse
doctors
    competence to treat alcoholism, 99,
        106, 136, 170
    diagnosis by, 107, 124
    duty to question, 71, 77
    examination by, 6, 109
    and psychotherapy, 117–21, 124
    reluctance to diagnose alcoholism,
        5, 16, 153
Drinking Sensibly (DHSS), 157
driving ability, 10, 11
    see also road accidents
drugs
    effect of, compared, 3–4, 20
    habit acquired, 90–91
    use of in treatment, 19, 110–15
drunkenness; see intoxication
Dutch courage, 67

earnings, 13, 86

see also employment
education, health, 129, 157, 160–61
Edwards, G., 143
effects of alcohol, 8–12
ego-alienation, 41
Emetine, 135
Employment
  aid to treatment, as, 140
  cooperation of workpeople, 116
  dismissal from, 88–9
  drink trade, in, 31, 34
  mortality tables, 156
  working efficiency, loss of, 85
  see also absenteeism
Emrick, C. D., 140–41
England
  consumption of drink in, 32
  drinking habits in, 36–7, 65
enzyme abnormalities, 62
epilepsy, alcoholic, 20, 92
Episcopalians, 35
escalation of drinking, 65–8
ethyl alcohol, 7
European Economic Community, 158
excessive drinkers
  defined, ix, 2
  dependancy circle of, 66–8
  psychology of, 35–6, 123
  stage of alcoholism, 80–83
  treatment of, effects of, 148

families of alcoholics, 93–105
  break up of, 89, 97
  children; *see* children
  cost of care of, 169
  effect on, 1, 43–4, 49–50, 168
  female, 102
  male, 93–102
  spouse; *see* spouse
  support from, 110, 140, 149–50
  treatment, involvement in, 99
  violence towards, 87
fathers of alcoholics, 44
fermentation, 7
Finland, 159
foetal alcohol syndrome, 27

food, alcohol as, 9
fortified wines, 8
France, 31
friends
  Alcoholics Anonymous, in, 133
  drinking, 73, 155
  loss of, 13, 46, 67, 83
  reaction of, 86
  re-establishment of after cure,
    147–9
  support from, 110, 140, 148
functional disorders, 23

gambling, 86
gastritis, 14
general practitioners; *see* doctors
Germany, 159
Glatt, M. M., 139
group behaviour, 30
group therapy, 117–21

habitual drinkers, 13
hallucinations, 17–19, 24–5
  see also delirium tremens
hangovers, 16
harm, physical
  chronic alcoholics, to, 91–2
  dependance, from, 66
  element in alcoholism, ix, 3–4,
    70–71, 80, 168
  excessive drinking, from, 83
Health Education Council, 160
Heminevrin, 111
heredity, 57, 62–4
hiding bottles, 89–90
home, drinking at, 74
homosexuality, 24, 42, 51–3
hormonal factors, 62
Horton, D., 30
hospitals
  abstinence in, 72
  admission rates, 156–7
  advice in, 92
  casualty departments, 128
  compulsory detention in, 23, 127
  out-patient treatment, 126–7, 143

hospitals – *contd.*
  preferable to prisons, 5
  recognition of alcoholism in, 107,
    124, 156
  remission after, 145
  treatment in, 126, 136
'host, environment, agent' theory,
  57–8, 110, 157
hostels, 129–30
hours of permitted sale, 60, 64, 158,
  169
hypnosis, 136

illness, recognition of alcoholism as,
  x, 5, 97–8, 105, 106, 107–8, 165
  by alcoholics themselves, 107
immature personalities, 47–9
impotence, sexual, 51
inability to abstain, 73
independence, apparent, of
  alcoholics, 43–6
inferiority, sense of, 45
inhibitions, release of, 9–11, 42, 53,
  intelligence, 21–2, 46
  see also brain
intoxication
  amount of alcohol required, ix
  chronic, 56
  daytime, 85
  dependance, and, 83
  effect of, 9
  recognition of, 13, 71–2
  society's view of, ix
  weekend, 88
  see also tolerance
isolation, 46, 67, 87, 89
  see also social problems
Italy, 31

James, William, 130
Jariwalla, A. G., 107
Jarman, C. M. B., 107
jaundice, 14
jealousy, 23, 88, 96, 150
Jellinek, E. M., 70, 146
Jews, 34–5, 65

Jung, Carl, 130

Kellett, J. M., 107
Korsakov psychosis, 20–22

Lavers, G. R., 34
Licensing Acts, 32, 37, 60, 64,
  158–9, 169
life expectancy, 155–6
liver
  cirrhosis of, 14, 31, 59, 71, 74, 92,
    145, 156, 160
  function of, 8
loss of control, 74, 85

Makella, K., 35
malnutrition, 13–15
marriage; *see* spouse
Medical Council on Alcoholism,
  170–71
medical examinations, 6, 109
  see also assessments; doctors
medical problem, alcoholism as, 5, 16
  see also illness
memory, loss of; *see* amnesia
Mental Health Acts, 127
mental illness; *see* brain
Methodists, 35
methods of drinking, 31–4
methylated spirits, 164
Mill, John Stuart, 158
money problems, 13, 86–7, 97
Mormons, 35
'morning after' feeling, 11
morning drinking, 73, 89
Moslems, 35, 65
mothers of alcoholics, 40, 42, 44, 48,
  93
motivation in treatment, 143

N1 factor, 62
National Council on Alcoholism, 34
nausea, 13, 14, 16
  as therapy, 134–5
nervous systems, 9–11, 15
neuroses, 54–5, 76, 79

Northern Ireland, 34
nurses, role of, 123

offence of drunkenness, 50
    see also crime; prison
Office of Health Economics, 154
opening hours; *see under* public
        houses
Orford, J., 143
Ötinger, Friedrich, 130
outlets for purchase of alcohol, 64,
        158–9
    see also public houses
Owens, E. P., 107
Oxford Group, 130
oxidation, 8–9

pancreatitis, 15
paranoid shift, 23–4, 45, 87–8
    see also self-pity
parents
    daughters' relations with, 93
    inheritance of alcoholism from,
        63–4, 65
    effect of alcoholism of, on children,
        103–5
    see also children; families; fathers;
        mothers
passive-aggressiveness, 103
passivity of alcoholics, 43
    see also dependence
pathological drinking, 33, 79
patterns, drinking, of alcoholics,
        70–79
pedestrians, drunken, 162
Pendery, M. L., 142
periodic alcoholism, 78–9
peripheral neuritis, 15, 71, 92
personality of alcoholics, ix, 38–56
physical attributes of alcoholics, 61–4
pituitary gland, 9
poison, alcohol as, 75
power, sense of, 42
predisposition to alcoholism, ix
pregnancy, 27–8

*Prevention and Health: Everyone's
    Business* (DHSS), 157
prevention of alcoholism, 61, 153,
        157–69
price of alcohol, 60–61, 64, 158, 169
prison
    lack of rehabilitation in, 5, 166
    remission after, 145
    see also assessment; crime
'problem drinkers', 6
prohibition (USA), 34
proof spirit, 8
proteins, 13
psychiatric units, x, 100
    see also hospitals
psychiatrists, 124–5, 136
psychoanalysts, 24
psychologists, clinical, 122–3
psychopathy, 41–2
psychoses, 79, 92, 126
psychotherapy, 58, 117–21, 139
public health aspects of alcoholism,
        153–7
public houses
    atmosphere of, 33–4
    drunkenness in, 159
    food in, 13
    opening hours, 60, 64
    women in, 33
    see also Licensing Acts

quantity of alcohol
    as cause of alcoholism, 57–61
    needed to intoxicate, ix
    see also availability

recognition of problem by
        alcoholics, 2, 107
    see also illness
recognition of alcoholism, 13, 71–2
    see also doctors; hospitals
recovery from drinking, rate of, 9
    see also 'safe limits'
rehabilitation after cure, 147–9
relations with others; *see* social
        problems

remission after abstinence, 2, 16, 72, 138–44
  likelihood of, 145
  not total disaster, 122
  prevention of, 111–15
  rates of, 143–4
  social drinking, to, 114, 139, 141–2, 148
remorse, 86–8
research required, 167–8
restrained alcoholics, 72–4
reversion; see remission
road accidents, x, 5, 59, 162–4, 169
  see also 'safe limits'
Roman Catholics, 35, 65
Royal College of Psychiatrists, 154, 161

'safe limits', 12, 65, 154, 161
Salvation Army, 165–6, 170
schizophrenia, 24, 25, 46
  alcoholism as symptom of, 76
Scotland
  drinking habits, in 33–4, 65, 154–5, 157
  opening hours in, 64, 159
Seebohm Rowntree, B., 34
self-confidence, lack of, 39
self-esteem, lack of, 43, 86, 117
  recovery of, 121
self-indulgence, 40, 43, 47, 49–51
self-pity, 87–8, 95
  see also paranoid shift
self-punishment, 53
'Serenity' (AA), 132
sexual problems, 51–3
  after cure, 150
  deviants, 51–2
  fear of sex, 51
  lack of drive, 51, 88
  spouse repulsed, 96
'shakes, the' (tremulousness), 17–18, 24, 89, 110
shelters in cities, 129
Silkworth, W. D., 130

skid rows, 5, 164–5
Sobell, M. B., and I. C., 142
social drinking
  acceptance of, ix–x, 3, 35, 42, 162
  alcoholism, leading to, 58
  distinguished from exessive, ix, 2
  gastritis from, 14
  Jewish approval of, 35
  limits of, 10–11
  pregnancy, during, 28
  return to after abstinence, 114, 139, 141–2, 148
social problems of alcoholics
  as cause of alcoholism, 63
  compulsive alcoholics, 75–6
  disruption, 1, 16, 36, 40–41, 45–6, 67
  exacerbate drinking, 86
  family affected by, 95–6
  friends, re-establishment of, 147–9
  improvement of, 39, 55
  isolation, 46, 67, 87, 89
  psycopathy, 41–2
  restrictions, 83, 85–6
  spouse, 100
social workers
  ability to treat alcoholics, 99, 106–7, 136, 139, 143, 150, 170
  psychotherapists, 117, 123
  types of help from, 115–16
society and drinking, 29–37, 65
sociopathy, 41–2
solitary drinkers, 39, 73–4
spirits
  alcohol content of, 8
  amount drunk, 32
  taxation of, 37
spouses
  behaviour pattern of, 93
  breakdown of marriage, 13, 87, 89, 97–100
  capability of, 95, 102, 103
  choice of by alcoholics, 93–4
  cure, problems after, 149–50
  deception of, 87
  head of household, as, 87, 149

help in treatment, 115, 149–50
illness of, 101
money problems of, 95
reforming influence of, 94
violence towards, 87
stages of alcoholism, 80–92
stimulant, fallacy of alcohol as, 10
stress, 54–5
escape from, 57
see also neuroses
suicide, 26, 72, 90–91, 126
supermarket sales of alcohol, 33
supplies of drink; see availability
symptomatic alcoholism, 76–8, 148

taxation of alcohol, 158
teenage drunkenness, 37
see also age of drinkers
teetotallers; see abstinence
temperance movement, 37
tension, reduced by alcohol, ix,
    29–30, 82–3
tolerance levels, 4, 12, 71, 83
lowering of, 91–2, 168
'Traditional' (AA), 131–2
traffic accidents; see road accidents
treatment, 106–37
absence of, 141
abstinence, during, 152
agencies, 99
availability of, 108, 167
family involvement in, 99
non-medical, 5: see also social
    workers
plans, 108–37
principles of, 69
psychotherapy, 58
rates of admission for, 156–7
requirements of alcoholics, 2, 4
results of, 138–44

studies, 169–70
units, 125, 129, 156, 170
Trevelyan, G. M., 36
tremulousness; see 'shakes, the'
Twelve Steps (AA), 131, 146

ulcers, gastric, 71, 72
unemployment, 37, 94
United States of America, 34
urine, 9

violence, 43, 45
towards spouses, 23, 87, 96
vitamins, 20, 116
B, 13, 15, 22

weekend drunkenness, 88
Wernicke's encephalopathy, 22
Wilson, W. D., 130
wine, 7–8
withdrawal symptoms, 2, 19, 20, 73,
    75, 168
cause of, 16–17
compared with drug addicts, 4
detoxification, with, 110–11, 128
treatment after, 122, 136
treatment of, 126
see also delirium tremens
women drinkers
cirrhosis, high risk of, 14
consumption by, 5, 65
habits, 155, 168
psychology of, 44–5
public houses, in, 33
'safe limits' for, 154, 161
secret, 74
success in treatment of, 140
World Health Organization, 3, 4, 153
Wormwood Scrubs, 166

READ MORE IN PENGUIN

In every corner of the world, on every subject under the sun, Penguin represents quality and variety – the very best in publishing today.

For complete information about books available from Penguin – including Puffins, Penguin Classics and Arkana – and how to order them, write to us at the appropriate address below. Please note that for copyright reasons the selection of books varies from country to country.

In the United Kingdom: Please write to *Dept. JC, Penguin Books Ltd, FREEPOST, West Drayton, Middlesex UB7 0BR*

If you have any difficulty in obtaining a title, please send your order with the correct money, plus ten per cent for postage and packaging, to *PO Box No. 11, West Drayton, Middlesex UB7 0BR*

In the United States: Please write to *Penguin USA Inc., 375 Hudson Street, New York, NY 10014*

In Canada: Please write to *Penguin Books Canada Ltd, 10 Alcorn Avenue, Suite 300, Toronto, Ontario M4V 3B2*

In Australia: Please write to *Penguin Books Australia Ltd, 487 Maroondah Highway, Ringwood, Victoria 3134*

In New Zealand: Please write to *Penguin Books (NZ) Ltd, 182–190 Wairau Road, Private Bag, Takapuna, Auckland 9*

In India: Please write to *Penguin Books India Pvt Ltd, 706 Eros Apartments, 56 Nehru Place, New Delhi 110 019*

In the Netherlands: Please write to *Penguin Books Netherlands B.V., Keizersgracht 231 NL–1016 DV Amsterdam*

In Germany: Please write to *Penguin Books Deutschland GmbH, Friedrichstrasse 10–12, W–6000 Frankfurt/Main 1*

In Spain: Please write to *Penguin Books S. A., C. San Bernardo 117–6° E–28015 Madrid*

In Italy: Please write to *Penguin Italia s.r.l., Via Felice Casati 20, I–20124 Milano*

In France: Please write to *Penguin France S. A., 17 rue Lejeune, F–31000 Toulouse*

In Japan: Please write to *Penguin Books Japan, Ishikiribashi Building, 2–5–4, Suido, Tokyo 112*

In Greece: Please write to *Penguin Hellas Ltd, Dimocritou 3, GR–106 71 Athens*

In South Africa: Please write to *Longman Penguin Southern Africa (Pty) Ltd, Private Bag X08, Bertsham 2013*